T0215834

Fast Facts About **NEUROCRITICAL CARE**: A Quick Reference for the Advanced Practice Provider *(McLaughlin)*

Fast Facts for the **NEW NURSE PRACTITIONER**: What You Really Need to Know, Second Edition *(Aktan)*

Fast Facts for **NURSE PRACTITIONERS:** Practice Essentials for Clinical Subspecialties *(Aktan)*

Fast Facts for the **NURSE PRECEPTOR**: Keys to Providing a Successful Preceptorship *(Ciocco)*

Fast Facts for the **NURSE PSYCHOTHERAPIST**: The Process of Becoming *(Jones, Tusaie)*

Fast Facts About **NURSING AND THE LAW**: Law for Nurses *(Grant, Ballard)*

Fast Facts About the **NURSING PROFESSION**: Historical Perspectives *(Hunt)*

Fast Facts for the **OPERATING ROOM NURSE**: An Orientation and Care Guide, Second Edition *(Criscitelli)*

Fast Facts for the **PEDIATRIC NURSE**: An Orientation Guide *(Rupert, Young)*

Fast Facts Handbook for **PEDIATRIC PRIMARY CARE:** A Guide for Nurse Practitioners and Physician Assistants *(Ruggiero, Ruggiero)*

Fast Facts About **PRESSURE ULCER CARE FOR NURSES**: How to Prevent, Detect, and Resolve Them *(Dziedzic)*

Fast Facts About **PTSD**: A Guide for Nurses and Other Health Care Professionals *(Adams)*

Fast Facts for the **RADIOLOGY NURSE**: An Orientation and Nursing Care Guide, Second Edition *(Grossman)*

Fast Facts About **RELIGION FOR NURSES**: Implications for Patient Care *(Taylor)*

Fast Facts for the **SCHOOL NURSE**: What You Need to Know, Third Edition *(Loschiavo)*

Fast Facts About **SEXUALLY TRANSMITTED INFECTIONS**: A Nurse's Guide to Expert Patient Care *(Scannell)*

Fast Facts for **STROKE CARE NURSING**: An Expert Care Guide, Second Edition *(Morrison)*

Fast Facts for the **STUDENT NURSE**: Nursing Student Success *(Stabler-Haas)*

Fast Facts About **SUBSTANCE USE DISORDERS**: What Every Nurse, APRN, and PA Needs to Know *(Marshall, Spencer)*

Fast Facts for the **TRAVEL NURSE**: Travel Nursing *(Landrum)*

Fast Facts for the **TRIAGE NURSE**: An Orientation and Care Guide, Second Edition *(Visser, Montejano)*

Fast Facts for the **WOUND CARE NURSE**: Practical Wound Management *(Kifer)*

Fast Facts for **WRITING THE DNP PROJECT**: Effective Structure, Content, and Presentation *(Christenbery)*

Forthcoming FAST FACTS Books

Fast Facts for the **ADULT-GERONTOLOGY ACUTE CARE NURSE PRACTITIONER** *(Carpenter)*

Fast Facts for **CREATING A SUCCESSFUL TELEHEALTH SERVICE**: A How-to Guide for Nurse Practitioners *(Heidesch)*

Fast Facts About **DIVERSITY, EQUITY, AND INCLUSION** *(Davis)*

Fast Facts for the **ER NURSE**: Guide to a Successful Emergency Department Orientation, Fourth Edition *(Buettner)*

Fast Facts for the **L&D NURSE**: Labor & Delivery Orientation, Third Edition *(Groll)*

Fast Facts About **LGBTQ CARE FOR NURSES** *(Traister)*

Fast Facts for the **NEONATAL NURSE**: Care Essentials for Normal and High-Risk Neonates, Second Edition *(Davidson)*

Fast Facts for the **NURSE PRECEPTOR**: Keys to Providing a Successful Preceptorship, Second Edition *(Ciocco)*

Fast Facts for **PATIENT SAFETY IN NURSING** *(Hunt)*

Visit www.springerpub.com to order.

FAST FACTS About
COMPETENCY-BASED EDUCATION IN NURSING

Ruth A. Wittmann-Price, PHD, RN, CNS, CNE, CHSE, CNEcl, ANEF, FAAN, is the undergraduate chair of nursing for Thomas Jefferson University, College of Nursing in Center City, Philadelphia. She received her BSN degree from Felician College in Lodi, New Jersey; her master's from Columbia University, New York City; and completed her PhD in nursing at Widener University, Chester, Pennsylvania. Dr. Wittmann-Price's PhD received the Dean's Award for Excellence. She developed a mid-range nursing theory entitled "Emancipated Decision-Making (EDM) in Women's Health Care" and has tested her theory in four studies. The EDM theory recognizes that oppression continues to exist in the healthcare setting and is imposed by society for purposes of situational control affecting the decisions women make about healthcare for themselves and their families. The EDM theory is referenced in multiple books and is being used in Thailand, South Africa, Brazil, Colombia, the United Kingdom, and Canada. The University of Limpopo, in South Africa, has applied the theory to the Community-Oriented Nursing Education Program for Women and Child Health project. This project institutes a community-oriented nursing education program to improve the health of women and children. Dr. Wittmann-Price has secured over $6 million in federal funding to support disadvantaged nursing students to care for patients in medically underserved communities. Dr. Wittmann-Price has authored over 16 books, numerous articles, and presents internationally and nationally.

Karen K. Gittings, DNP, RN, CNE, CNEcl, Alumnus CCRN, is a professor of nursing and dean of the School of Health Sciences at Francis Marion University, Florence, South Carolina. Dr. Gittings received her diploma in nursing from The Washington Hospital School of Nursing, Washington, Pennsylvania and her BSN from the University of Maryland, Baltimore County campus. She earned her MSN with a specialization in nursing education and her DNP at Duquesne University in Pittsburgh, Pennsylvania. She was a 2015 to 2016 Amy V. Cockcroft Fellow, achieved certification in online instruction in 2011, became a certified nurse educator (CNE) in 2013, and earned certification as an academic clinical nurse educator (CNEcl) with the inaugural group of test-takers. Dr. Gittings has extensive experience in critical care nursing and has been a certified critical-care RN (CCRN) since 1991. Her areas of teaching and clinical expertise are medical–surgical nursing, critical care, and cardiac nursing. She has taught students across the curriculum in the BSN, MSN, and DNP programs. Dr. Gittings has co-authored two books and eight book chapters. Dr. Gittings has also presented nationally on multiple education-related topics. She is past president of Francis Marion University's chapter of Phi Kappa Phi, Chi Lambda Chapter of Sigma Theta Tau International and the Pee Dee Area Chapter of the American Association of Critical Care Nurses. She is a recipient of multiple Outstanding Faculty Teaching Awards at Francis Marion University and the South Carolina Palmetto Gold Award (2005).

FAST FACTS About
COMPETENCY-BASED EDUCATION IN NURSING

How to Teach Competency Mastery

Ruth A. Wittmann-Price, PhD, RN, CNS, CNE, CHSE, CNEcl, ANEF, FAAN
Karen K. Gittings, DNP, RN, CNE, CNEcl, Alumnus CCRN

EDITORS

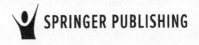 SPRINGER PUBLISHING

Springer Publishing Company, LLC
11 West 42nd Street, New York, NY 10036
www.springerpub.com
connect.springerpub.com/

Acquisitions Editor: Rachel X. Landes
Compositor: Amnet Systems

ISBN: 978-0-8261-3653-4
ebook ISBN: 978-0-8261-3663-3
DOI: 10.1891/9780826136633

20 21 22 / 5 4 3 2 1

The author and the publisher of this Work have made every effort to use sources believed to be reliable to provide information that is accurate and compatible with the standards generally accepted at the time of publication. Because medical science is continually advancing, our knowledge base continues to expand. Therefore, as new information becomes available, changes in procedures become necessary. We recommend that the reader always consult current research and specific institutional policies before performing any clinical procedure or delivering any medication. The author and publisher shall not be liable for any special, consequential, or exemplary damages resulting, in whole or in part, from the readers' use of, or reliance on, the information contained in this book. The publisher has no responsibility for the persistence or accuracy of URLs for external or third-party Internet websites referred to in this publication and does not guarantee that any content on such websites is, or will remain, accurate or appropriate.

Library of Congress Cataloging-in-Publication Data

Names: Wittmann-Price, Ruth A., editor. | Gittings, Karen K., editor.
Title: Fast facts about competency-based education in nursing : how to teach competency mastery / [edited by] Ruth A. Wittmann-Price, Karen K. Gittings.
Other titles: Fast facts (Springer Publishing Company)
Description: New York, NY : Springer Publishing Company, LLC, [2021] | Series: Fast facts | Includes bibliographical references and index. |
Identifiers: LCCN 2020035394 (print) | LCCN 2020035395 (ebook) | ISBN 9780826136534 (paperback) | ISBN 9780826136633 (ebook)
Subjects: MESH: Education, Nursing | Competency-Based Education | Professional Competence—standards | Educational Measurement—standards
Classification: LCC RT71 (print) | LCC RT71 (ebook) | NLM WY 18 | DDC 610.73071—dc23
LC record available at https://lccn.loc.gov/2020035394
LC ebook record available at https://lccn.loc.gov/2020035395

Contact us to receive discount rates on bulk purchases.
We can also customize our books to meet your needs.
For more information please contact: sales@springerpub.com

Publisher's Note: New and used products purchased from third-party sellers are not guaranteed for quality, authenticity, or access to any included digital components.

Printed in the United States of America.

To my grandchildren Alice, Henry, and Regina.
—Ruth A. Wittmann-Price

For my much-loved parents.
—Karen K. Gittings

Contents

Contributors

Tracy P. George, DNP, APRN-BC, CNE

Assistant Professor of Nursing
Department of Nursing
Francis Marion University
Florence, South Carolina

Karen K. Gittings, DNP, RN, CNE, CNEcl, Alumnus CCRN

Professor of Nursing
Dean, School of Health Sciences
Francis Marion University
Florence, South Carolina

Dawn M. Goodolf, PhD, RN

Associate Professor
Chairperson, Department of Nursing
Moravian College
Bethlehem, Pennsylvania

Catherine Johnson, PhD, FNP, PNP

Clinical Associate Professor
School of Nursing
Duquesne University
Pittsburgh, Pennsylvania

Evelyn (Evie) Lengetti, PhD, RN-BC

Assistant Professor of Nursing
Assistant Dean, Continuing Education
Villanova University
Villanova, Pennsylvania

Denise Lucas, PhD, FNP-BC, CRNP, FAANP

Clinical Associate Professor
Chair, Advanced Practice Programs
School of Nursing
Duquesne University
Pittsburgh, Pennsylvania

Rev. Robert G. Mulligan, OSFS, MA, MEd

Chaplain—Campus Ministry
Instructor of Education—Center for Education, Advocacy,
    and Social Justice
Chestnut Hill College
Philadelphia, Pennsylvania

Tiffany A. Phillips, DNP, NP-C

Assistant Professor of Nursing
Department of Nursing
Francis Marion University
Florence, South Carolina

Ruth A. Wittmann-Price, PhD, RN, CNS, CNE, CNEcl, CHSE, ANEF, FAAN

Professor of Nursing
Chair, Undergraduate Programs, Center City
Jefferson College of Nursing
Thomas Jefferson University
Philadelphia, Pennsylvania

Foreword

The case for competency-based nursing education has been raised by our clinical practice partners for many years. We know that competency is vital to patient safety with respect to nursing practice. The bottom line is that no one will argue with the fact that we want or need competent nurses. New graduate nurses and advanced practice nurses need specific, entry-level skills to function in the clinical setting. Competence has traditionally been defined as functional adequacy and the ability to integrate knowledge, skills, attitudes, and values with practice (Meretoja & Koponen, 2012). The National Council of State Boards of Nursing (2005) describes competency as the ability to apply knowledge and interpersonal, decision-making, and psychomotor skills to nursing practice roles.

We sometimes hear that new nurses are not prepared for the realities of practice or cannot assume a full assignment independently. As we proceed down the competency-based education path, which I support, I believe we need to do so with a degree of caution. Novice nurses and advanced practice nurses still need a comprehensive orientation and associated supports. A competency-based education is not a quick fix to onboard nurses or a substitution for a liberal arts education. When we think of the robust orientation of a new attorney or accountant, they are not assigned to the high-profile critical cases or biggest clients fresh out of school; however, nurses are often called to care for critically ill patients less than three months or six months on the job post-graduation. Competency-based education is a valid way to evaluate safe nursing practice, especially with respect to certain high-risk skills, but not a replacement for a relevant, supportive orientation.

In 1998, Dr. Michael Dreher and I developed Drexel University's BSN curriculum. We decided to offer a capstone course, called Senior Seminar. Before students could graduate, they needed to pass a standardized comprehensive exam, pass a final complex standardized patient exam, and successfully demonstrate 10 core critical nursing skills in the last semester. At the time, we did not have access to the body of research available today that supports simulation as a means to assess nurses' skill in detecting high-risk changes in patients or that practicing active retrieval of knowledge enhances student performance on meaningful assessments and improves long-term meaningful learning (Karpicke, 2012). We were definitely united in our respective professional opinions that working without adequate knowledge and competence was harmful to patients and, in our view, unethical. We also used competency-based education to teach technology skills necessary to access and evaluate patient information at the point-of-care.

Meaningful learning is thought to produce organized, coherent, and integrated mental models that allow students to make inferences and apply knowledge necessary for the nursing discipline so they can practice safely. Competency-based education is not new. It provides an avenue to promote institutional accountability, address employer concerns, and assist with student transfer of knowledge and skills. Should the *entire* curriculum be competency-based? There is real value in teaching students how to think, write, speak, debate, and so on. Not every subject can or should be competency-based.

We should use our best judgment as to when competency-based education applies.

Mary Ellen Smith Glasgow, PhD, RN, ANEF, FAAN
Dean and Professor
Duquesne University

REFERENCES

Karpicke, J. D. (2012). Retrieval-based learning: Active retrieval promotes meaningful learning. *Current Directions in Psychological Science, 21*(3), 157–163. https://doi.org/10.1177/0963721412443552

Meretoja, R., & Koppnen, L. (2012). A systematic model to compare nurses' optimal and actual competencies in the clinical setting. *Journal of Advanced Nursing, 68*(2), 414–422. https://doi.org/10.1111/j.1365-2648.2011.05754.x

National Council of State Boards of Nursing. (2005). *Meeting the ongoing challenge of continued competence*.

Preface

With the move toward assuring the public that nursing students are graduating with the needed competencies to step into their very important careers, competency-based education (CBE) has become increasingly important. This *Fast Facts* book describes how competence is the outcome and how nursing students can rise to meet the cognitive, psychomotor, and affective skills needed to become professional nurses who make a positive impact on the health of individuals, families, and communities.

The novel coronavirus (COVID-19) crisis has underscored the importance of CBE. Nurse educators throughout the country have analyzed standards, criteria, regulations, and student learning outcomes to define the competencies needed during this disruptive time in nursing education. Nurse educators have creatively and innovatively assisted nursing students to meet the needed competencies in alternative formats, thereby ensuring graduates will have the cognitive, psychomotor, and affective skills needed to become excellent professional nurses.

This *Fast Facts* book is arranged to assist nurse educators in understanding and reflecting on the concepts and components of CBE, as well as the pragmatic implementation of CBE. Chapter 1 provides an overview of CBE, including the major tenets. This chapter also provides the history of CBE and discusses its goals and meaning for students.

Chapter 2 demonstrates how CBE can be infused into a nursing curriculum complete with an organizing framework. This chapter demonstrates how courses fit a CBE framework and how CBE aligns with student learning outcomes. Chapter 2 also discusses the methods used in CBE to ensure student success through built-in remediation processes.

Chapter 3 delves further into the practice of writing measurable competencies. The original and useful Competency Outcomes and Performance Assessment (COPA) Model is outlined as a template that ensures that CBE meets the goals of the nursing program. Chapter 3 also discusses the difference between a competency statement and an objective. Also, importantly, this chapter looks at how different learning styles thrive in a CBE learning environment.

Chapter 4 explains to nurse educators the mechanisms for developing CBE assessments. The three learning domains and their relation to CBE are outlined and the need for validated assessments are emphasized. Valid and reliable assessments are being developed in all three learning domains and examples are provided.

Chapter 5 discusses the evaluation of student competencies. Review of how evaluation in all three learning domains is completed and how the domains can be broken down into practical learning goals is demonstrated. The evaluation process for CBE is the culmination of an integrated CBE program and highlights how students can successfully meet needed nursing competencies.

Chapter 6 demonstrates the important aspect of continuous process improvement. All nurse educators understand that no program implementation is ever complete. In order to meet students' learning needs in the best method possible, the process goes through continuous evaluation. Chapter 6 outlines succinct and effective process improvement methods to continuously improve a CBE curriculum.

Chapters 7 through 9 demonstrate how CBE can be adjusted to each nursing educational level—baccalaureate (BSN), master's (MSN), and doctor of nursing practice (DNP). These chapters discuss standards for each educational level and how to apply those professional standards to CBE methodologies. Chapter 7 discusses CBE and its relevance to undergraduate nursing education and how to apply CBE to active learning strategies in undergraduate curricula. Chapter 8 applies CBE concepts to the standards and regulations of MSN degrees, and Chapter 9 outlines the competencies needed to achieve a doctor of nursing practice degree and make system healthcare changes. These three final chapters help with the specific implementation of CBE and provide examples and suggestions.

This *Fast Facts* book is a clear, succinct tool needed by nurse educators to move from a traditional nursing curriculum to one that ensures that nursing students are ready for today's healthcare challenges. Events that disrupt nursing education, such as the COVID-19 crisis, can be more easily overcome if the achievement of competencies is the focus and when nurses continue to develop creative and innovative methods to ensure needed competencies are met. This *Fast Facts* format uses examples and evidence to assist nurse educators to take the first steps in moving a nursing program toward a CBE and ensuring nursing graduates are ready to face evolving healthcare needs and future events.

Ruth Wittmann-Price
Karen K. Gittings

1

Overview of Competency-Based Education (CBE)

Ruth A. Wittmann-Price

"You don't have to be great to start, but you have to start to be great."

— Zig Ziglar

OBJECTIVES

- Describe the components of competency-based education (CBE).
- Discuss the goals of CBE.
- Compare the development of CBE to the current educational social mandates.

INTRODUCTION

Today's healthcare environment increasingly calls for more positive and efficient outcomes. The 1999 Institute of Medicine (IOM) report "To Err is Human" underscored the need for better patient outcomes due to the estimated 98,000 deaths per year made by healthcare errors (Institute of Medicine Committee on Quality of Health Care in America, 2000). Nurses understand that positive patient/ client care outcomes occur when interventions are based on best practices, and best practices are developed and nurtured during the educational processes for healthcare professionals.

Much literature has been written about the education-to-practice gap (Leggett, 2015) and, without changes in education, that gap will only widen. After all, healthcare is becoming ever-increasingly complicated due to technology, the aging population, reimbursement, longer lifespans that include people with chronic and complex healthcare issues, and other variables. Many healthcare organizations have developed "residency" programs to close that education-to-practice gap.

Competency-based education (CBE) is academia's solution to decrease the ever-growing education-to-practice gap. CBE is outcomes-based and can improve healthcare quality (Sargeant et al., 2018). The goal of healthcare education is to graduate competent and caring providers. CBE, specifically, assists professional nurses in providing quality healthcare that is based on evidence to promote best practice (Figure 1.1).

Five Characteristics of Competencies

1. Focus on the performance of the end-product or instructional goal
2. Reflect what is learned in the instructional program
3. Are expressed in terms of measurable behavior
4. Are used as a standard for judging competence independent of others' performance
5. Inform learners and other stakeholders about what is expected of them (Covert et al., 2019).

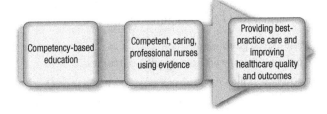

Figure 1.1 Competency-based education.

COMPETENCY-BASED EDUCATION

CBE is defined by Sargeant et al. (2018) as "An outcomes-based approach to the design, implementation, assessment, and evaluation of education programs using an organizing framework of competencies" (p. 128).

Four Essential Components of CBE

1. Curriculum design is based on abilities or competencies
2. CBE is focused on outcomes that can be assessed by multiple evaluation methods (Sargeant et al., 2018)
3. CBE is learner-centered and congruent with constructivism, in which students understand the educational goals and independently construct knowledge themselves to reach the goals
4. CBE is responsive to society because graduates have the skills needed as practicing professional nurses (Wittmann-Price et al., 2017).

Fast Facts

CBE's goal is to prepare nursing students for real-world practice. CBE is being driven by stakeholders who are finding that healthcare graduates lack readiness for their roles (Storrar et al., 2019).

Past educational models have emphasized components that are not elements of CBE, including:

- Time-based goals
- Content coverage without specific outcomes (Gruppen et al., 2016).

In CBE, nursing students are encouraged to work at their own pace to attain the abilities and skills needed for their profession. The responsibility of mastering skills is placed on the student, promoting student accountability. Learning is more flexible than it has been in the past (Touchie & Cate, 2016).

CBE builds the learning and the curriculum around competencies needed for the professional setting. Competencies are not just hands-on nursing skills; they include knowledge and professional attitude. Professional attributes must include all three domains of learning, or they will not meet the demands of professional nursing (Robinson, 2018). CBE encourages "mastery of skills" (Leggett, 2015, p. 108) by building on cognitive knowledge and professionalism and applying it in the clinical setting (Leggett, 2015).

Fast Facts

Although CBE is outcomes-based, the process is still important to infuse inclusion and content, and allow for exploration of special interests (Storrar et al., 2019).

BOX 1.1 EVIDENCE-BASED TEACHING PRACTICE

Mace and Bacon (2018) surveyed athletic trainers ($n = 163$) to find out how much they know about CBE and how confident they were in using it as an educational modality. Knowledge and confidence scores were both low, demonstrating that although the term CBE is used in the discipline, faculty needed further information.

SYNONYMS AND DEFINITIONS FOR CBE

Medical education has coined the term "competency-based medical education (CBME),"while undergraduate psychology refers to competencies needed by graduates as "entrustable professional activities" (Grus & Rozensky, 2019). Other authors have referred to CBE as developing "practice-specific competencies" (Sargeant et al., 2018).

Several healthcare organizations and authors have defined and differentiated between the words "competence" and "competency." These definitions provide nursing faculty with guidance and understanding for curriculum development (Table 1.1).

Table 1.1

Definitions of Competence and Competency		
	Competence	Competency
Medical Education	Competence is abilities that are on a continuum and can include all learning domains appropriate to the content. Competence has to be described with qualifiers in order to properly understand the learner's stage. A learner's competence will change at different times in their career and in different settings (Frank et al., 2010).	A learner can demonstrate competency by an observable skill through cognitive reasoning, psychomotor ability, or affective behavior. Competency can be measured through evaluation techniques and can be staged depending on the level of the learner (Frank et al., 2010).
The American Nurses Credentialing Center	Competence is more than the here and now; it also includes a learner's potential (ANCC, 2019).	

(continued)

Table 1.1

	Definitions of Competence and Competency (*continued*)	
	Competence	**Competency**
The American Nurses Association		Competency in nursing care can be measured, includes all learning domains, and is based on evidence and standards of practice (ANA, 2015).
Higher Education		Competency is more than knowledge and includes the application of knowledge required by a profession (Bushway et al., 2018).
American Registry of Radiologic Technologists	Performance that is effective and up to standard and can be done consistently (ARRT, 2014).	
Nursing Education		Students are able to understand knowledge and use it in the care of patients, to evaluate their care, and to make adjustments to improve outcomes (Anema & McCoy, 2010).

Source: Adapted from American Nurses Association. (2015). *Nursing: Scope and standards of practice* (3rd ed.), p. 86; American Nurses Credentialing Center. (2019). *Awarding credit for outcome based professional development: Outcomes based-CE model manual*, p. 10; American Registry of Radiology Technologists. (2014). *Competency*. https://www.jrcert.org/resources/governance/accreditation-policies/11-400/, p. 2; Anema, M. G., & McCoy, J. (2010). *Competency-based nursing education: A guide to achieving outstanding learning outcomes*. Springer Publishing Company; Bushway, B., Dodge, L., & Long, C. (2018). *A leader's guide to competency-based education: From inception to implementation*. Stylus, p. 1; Frank, J. R., Snell, L. S., Cate, O. T., Holmboe, E. S., Carraccio, C., Swing, S. R., Harris, P., Glasgow, N. J., Campbell, C., Dath, D., Harden, R. M., Lobst, W., Long, D. M., Mungroo, R., Richardson, D. L., Sherbino, J., Silver, I., Taber, S., Talbot, M., & Harris, K. A. (2010). Competency-based medical education: Theory to practice. *Medical Teacher, 32*, 638–645. http://dx.doi.org/10.1080/0142159X.2017.1315069, p. 624.

Critical competencies are competencies that must be internalized by every nursing graduate, such as patient identification. *Core competencies* usually mean the foundational competencies needed for a profession. Both critical and core competencies are derived from expert opinion and evidence-based practice (EBP).

The following definitions of *"outcome"* underscore that the outcome is the end product nurse educators (academic or clinical) would like to see when observing or assessing students or staff.

The ANCC (2019, p. 4) defines an outcome as "a specific and quantifiable variable by which attainment of objectives may be judged." Additionally, Bennett et al. (2017) define *"expertise"* as the possession of expert skill or knowledge in a particular field that allows one to proficiently perform tasks. Expertise should lead to *"quality care,"* which Bennett and colleagues define as "an aim that increases the likelihood of desirable and consistent health outcomes with current knowledge within a given profession" (p. 98).

HISTORY OF COMPETENCY-BASED EDUCATION

Medical education was one of the first professions to adopt CBE over 50 years ago (Mace & Bacon, 2018). CBME traces its roots back to 1978 when McGaghie et al. (1978) at the US Accreditation Council for Graduate Medical Education recommended: "The intended outcome is a health-professional who can practice at a defined level of proficiency, in accord with local conditions, to meet local needs" (p. 18).

The psychology profession has used CBE proficiently on a graduate educational level for approximately 30+ years. Psychologists developed a competency cube and identified foundational competencies in ethics and diversity, and functional competencies in assessment and intervention. After the competency cube development, psychologists developed benchmarks and descriptors to assist educators in assessing graduate students' achievements. The competency descriptors included:

- Readiness for practicum
- Readiness for internship
- Readiness for practice
  (Grus & Rozensky, 2019).

CBE requires ongoing research to continuously identify the best practices to know what competencies are critical and how those competencies should be implemented (Gruppen et al., 2017). It makes perfect sense that CBE has grown out of the EBP era in nursing.

Fast Facts

CBE is being used effectively by healthcare organizations' professional development departments. Sargeant et al. (2018) state, "competency-based professional development is envisioned to place health needs and patient outcomes at the center" (p. 125).

DRIVING FORCES

Changes occur in healthcare curricula much more rapidly due to increases in scientific knowledge and more sophisticated technology. In the past, more generalist knowledge defined practitioners, but with increasing specialties, generalist knowledge is no longer sufficient (Touchie & Cate, 2016). CBE is diversified enough to include specific competencies for specialties (Grus & Rozensky, 2019).

Fast Facts

The goal of CBE is "moving the learner from one place to another" (Shinner & Graebe, 2019, p. 102).

As part of a larger push to align didactic content to real-world experience, CBE has expanded from health sciences into liberal arts curricula. This paradigm shift occurred partly because of the 2013 governmental policy "Making College Affordable: A Better Agenda for the Middle Class." CBE enhances education quality because applicability is the goal (Leggett, 2015).

Nursing advisory boards are essential in developing and maintaining a CBE curriculum. Advisory groups are stakeholders, such as employers and graduates who are ideal candidates to relay what current competencies are needed in the field. Curricula changes should be based on the real-world activities and competencies needed by the professional in the work environment to meet the needs of safe patient care (Leggett, 2015).

BOX 1.1 EVIDENCE-BASED TEACHING PRACTICE

Bennett et al. (2017) studied the education practice gap to identify competencies needed by graduate registered nurses ($n = 37$). The researchers found that the majority of respondents stated they did not acquire critically needed competencies when they were students.

OPPOSING FORCES

Authors have identified possible negative effects for students learning in a CBE curriculum, such as:

- Demotivation to learn further once a competency is attained
- A focus on minimal standards
- Increasing faculty and administrative workload since the timing of assessment is predicated on the individuality of the student
- Reducing needed content (Touchie & Cate, 2016)

- Some nurse educators may not be comfortable in providing student feedback about intrinsic characteristics such as:
  - Communication
  - Professionalism
  - Advocacy (Ferguson et al., 2017).

THEORETICAL UNDERPINNINGS OF CBE

CBE is an ongoing process, not a final achievement. CBE allows for continual refinement of student performance (Leggett, 2015) and takes into account the context of the competencies being taught and learned. Post-modern education rightly addresses the social influences placed upon graduates. CBE is rooted in objectives or competencies and is therefore akin to behaviorism (Touchie & Cate, 2016). Opponents of behaviorism claim human knowledge and understanding cannot be adequately predicted. CBE also has components of constructivism because the individual student is building knowledge in their own time frame (Dieklemann, 1997). Besides observable competencies, healthcare professionals need other skills that are difficult to assess by measurable objectives:

- Situational awareness
- Metacognition
- Balancing attentiveness and automaticity
- Interprofessional collaboration
  (Touchie & Cate, 2016).

For CBE to work, it must be integrated into all three domains of learning (cognitive, psychomotor, and affective)

Another outcome of CBE may be lower healthcare cost. By using best practices to define competencies and having future practitioners achieve competence, healthcare waste may ultimately be decreased. Theoretically, nursing implementation should be more effective using a CBE model (Kopf et al., 2018).

1.1 Example Vignette

A new faculty member is developing competencies and believes the competencies should be in her course to assist students in eventually achieving the final program competencies. The new faculty member is having difficulty distinguishing between a competency and a student learning outcome. The faculty mentor, a seasoned teacher, uses Gosselin (2019) to explain the difference:

- *A competency is a general statement that describes the desired knowledge, skills, and behaviors of a student graduating from a program (or completing a course). Competencies commonly define the applied skills and knowledge that enable people to successfully perform in professional, educational, and other life contexts.*

- *A student learning outcome is a very specific statement that describes exactly what a student will be able to do in some measurable way. There may be more than one measurable outcome defined for a given competency (p. 1).*

THE STUDENT INVOLVED IN COMPETENCY-BASED EDUCATION

Nursing students involved in CBE need to adapt an empowered stance. CBE requires two important learner attributes:

- Self-assessment
- Self-regulation

Although students may not always judge their self-assessments as accurately as needed, with proper feedback from a teacher, the student can learn where to focus their attention (Gruppen et al., 2017). Performance feedback will be addressed in depth in Chapter 4.

SUMMARY

CBE was developed in response to the healthcare education-to-practice gap identified by stakeholders and outcomes-based patient care called for by accrediting and regulatory agencies to reduce costly healthcare errors.

Fundamental Attributes of CBE

- Valid, achievable competencies
- Time for students to move through learning at their own pace
- Effective and available learning resources
- A curriculum map to guide the learning and placement of competencies
- Valid, reliable assessment tools (Leggett, 2015).

CBE has been used by medicine the longest but is gaining utilization and popularity with many health professions, including nursing. CBE is theoretically akin to both behaviorism and constructivism and promotes student responsibility and self-regulatory skills while setting educational goals. Curricula are developed around the identified student competencies and are assessed by nurse educators with valid and reliable tools. Student competency achievement provides data for curriculum revision and educational process improvement.

REFERENCES

American Nurses Association. (2015). *Nursing: Scope and standards of practice* (3rd ed.).

American Nurses Credentialing Center. (2019). *Awarding credit for outcome based professional development: Outcomes based-CE model manual.*

American Registry of Radiology Technologists. (2014). *Competency.* https://www.jrcert.org/resources/governance/accreditation-poli cies/11-400/

Anema, M. G., & McCoy, J. (2010). *Competency-based nursing education: A guide to achieving outstanding learning outcomes.* Springer Publishing Company.

Bennett, L. L., Grimsley, A., Grimsley, L., & Rodd, J. (2017). The gap between nursing education and clinical skills. *The Association of Black Nursing Faculty Journal, Fall 17,* 96–102.

Bushway, B., Dodge, L., & Long, C. (2018). *A leader's guide to competency-based education: From inception to implementation.* Stylus.

Covert, H., Sherman, M., Miner, K., & Lichtyeld, M. (2019). Core competencies and a workforce framework for community health workers: A model for advancing the profession. *American Journal of Public Health, 109*(2), 320–327. http://dx.doi.org/10.2105/AJPH.2018.304737

Dieklemann, N. L. (1997). Creating a new pedagogy for nursing. *Journal of Nursing Education, 26*(4), 147–148. https://doi.org/10.3928/0148-4834-19970401-03

Ferguson, P. C., Caverzagie, K. J., Nousiainen, M. T., & Snell, L. (2017). Changing the culture of medical training: An important step toward the implementation of competency-based medical education. *Medical Teacher, 39*(6), 599–602. http://dx.doi.org/10.1080/0142159X.2017.1315079

Frank, J. R., Snell, L. S., Cate, O. T., Holmboe, E. S., Carraccio, C., Swing, S. R., Harris, P., Glasgow, N. J., Campbell, C., Dath, D., Harden, R. M., Lobst, W., Long, D. M., Mungroo, R., Richardson, D. L., Sherbino, J., Silver, I., Taber, S., Talbot, M., & Harris, K. A. (2010). Competency-based medical education: Theory to practice. *Medical Teacher, 32,* 638–645. http://dx.doi.org/10.1080/0142159X.2017.1315069

Gosselin, D. (2019). *Competencies and learning outcomes.* Integrate: Interdisciplinary teaching about Earth for future sustainability. https://serc.carleton.edu/integrate/programs/workforceprep/competencies_and_LO.html

Gruppen, L. D., Burkhardt, J. C., Fitzgerald, J. T., Funnell, M., Haftel, H. M., Lypson, M. L., Mullan, P. B., Santen, S. A., Sheets, K. J., Stalburg, C. M., & Vasquez, J. A. (2016). Competency-based education: Programme design and challenges to implementation. *Medical Education, 50,* 532–539. http://dx.doi.org/10.1111/medu.12977

Gruppen, L. D., Frank, J. R., Lockyer, J., Ross, S., Bould. M. D., Harris, P., Bhanji, F., Hodges, B. D., Snell, L., & Cate, O. T. (2017). Toward a research agenda for competency-based medical education. *Medical Teacher, 39*(6), 623–630. http://dx.doi.org/10.1080/0142159X.2017.1315065

Grus, C. L., & Rozensky, R. H. (2019). Competency-based continuing education in health service psychology: Ensuring quality, recommendations for change. *Professional Psychology: Research and Practice, 50*(2), 106–112. http://dx.doi.org/10.1037/pro0000218

Institute of Medicine Committee on Quality of Health Care in America. (2000). *To err is human: Building a safer health system.* Academies Press. https://www.ncbi.nlm.nih.gov/pubmed/25077248

Kopf, R. S., Watts, P. I., Meyer, E. S., & Moss, J. A. (2018). A competency-based curriculum for critical care nurse practitioners' transition to practice. *American Journal of Critical Care, 27*(5), 398–406. http://dx.doi.org/10.4037/ajcc2018101

Leggett, T. (2015). Competency-based education: A brief overview. *Radiation Therapist, 24*(1), 107–110.

Mace, K. L., & Bacon, C. E. W. (2018). Athletic training educators' knowledge and confidence about competency-based education. *Athletic Training Education Journal, 13*(4), 302–308. http://dx.doi.org/10.4085/1304302

McGaghie, W. C., Miller, G. E., Sajid, A. W., & Telder, T. W. (1978). *Competency-based curriculum development in medical education—An introduction.* https://apps.who.int/iris/bitstream/handle/10665/39703/WHO_PHP_68.pdf;jsessionid=8B59C12E452C0A87C371BB8441EA4838?sequence=1

Robinson, F. P. (2018). Competency-based education: An innovative option for nurses. *American Nurse Today, 13*(10), 38–40.

Sargeant, J., Wong, B. M., & Campbell, C. M. (2018). CPD of the future: A partnership between quality improvement and competency-based education. *Medical Education, 52,* 125–135. http://dx.doi.org/10.1111/medu.13407

Shinner, J., & Graebe, J. (2019). Continuing professional development: Utilizing competency-based education and the American Nurses Credentialing Center Outcome-based Continuing Education Model. *The Journal of Continuing Education in Nursing, 50*(3), 100–102. http://dx.doi.org/10.3928/00220124-20190218-02

Storrar, N., Hope, D., & Cameron, H. (2019). Student perspective on outcomes ad process: Recommendations for implementing competency-based education. *Medical Teacher, 41*(2), 161–166. http://dx.doi.org/10.3928/00220124-20180517-02

Touchie, C., & Cate, O. (2016). The promise, perils, problems and progress of competency-based medical education. *Medial Education, 50*, 93–100. http://dx.doi.org/10.1111/medu.12839

Wittmann-Price, R. A., Godshall, M., & Wilson, L. (Eds.). (2017). *Certified Nurse Educator (CNE) review manual* (3rd ed.). Springer Publishing Company.

2

Competency-Based Curriculum Development

Ruth A. Wittmann-Price

"Life is a curriculum unique to every student."
—Joyce Rachelle

OBJECTIVES

- Discuss the development of competency-based education (CBE) curricula.
- Compare CBE to traditional curriculum models.
- Identify leadership attributes needed to develop or revise curricula.

INTRODUCTION

Competency-based education (CBE) is becoming the new curriculum model in healthcare for several reasons:

- Need for greater practitioner accountability
- Increased social expectations for quality care

- Need for educational systems that can readily adapt to change (Ferguson et al., 2017).

This chapter will delve into the specifics of revising or developing a nursing curriculum using a CBE model. Curriculum revision or development must consider many variables, including the educational mission, the competencies identified as needed, the framework, and the constraints encountered in traditional educational systems.

STEPS IN REVISING OR DEVELOPING A CBE NURSING CURRICULUM

Revising or developing a curriculum is a rewarding process that takes time, teamwork, thought processes, flexibility, and an openness to change and new ideas. Often, nurse educators undertaking this endeavor have themselves been educated in a traditional, content-driven paradigm, which effects the process (Ferguson et al., 2017).

Requirements for Curriculum Development

- Culture change and buy-in from constituents
  - Stakeholder input is necessary because "in today's educational climate, the value of education is measured against job marketability" (Boland, 2017, p. 1).
- A strong, knowledgeable leader to explain the benefits of change to faculty and articulate the vision of the final product.
- Resources like time, as faculty need time to be involved in a curriculum change or development process.
- An active and extensive communication so all faculty are informed as changes are voted on and take place.

Even one seemingly small curriculum change affects many variables such as:

- Course credits
- Faculty oversight
- Allocation of resources

- Teaching responsibilities
- Graduation requirements

Step 1: Revisit the Education Organization's and Department of Nursing's Mission

Collectively, the faculty group should be able to articulate how the proposed curriculum model fits within the mission of the educational organization and the nursing program. Table 2.1. demonstrates a side by side congruency table.

Step 2: Identify Program Outcomes (Goals and Objectives)

The nursing program's outcomes are integrated with the competencies needed for graduates. Nursing faculty, when revising or developing a curriculum, need to establish and agree on the competencies needed for real-world practice by

Table 2.1

Mission and Curriculum Model Congruency Table

Organizational Mission Elements	Program Mission Elements	Elements of a CBE Curriculum Model
University XX endeavors to educate students from the region (nationally, internationally).	The Department of Nursing provides excellent education to students from the region (nationally, internationally).	CBE provides an efficient, effective educational model.
University XX promotes innovative learning based on current evidence to a diverse population of students in a real-world setting.	The Department of Nursing strives to educate competent, caring professionals from diverse backgrounds who can provide care in today's complex healthcare setting.	CBE builds the curriculum around competencies that include not only skills, but also cognition and attitude. It is done on an individual student level to encompass diversity.

graduates. Variables that need to be considered when identifying the competencies graduates should achieve include:

- Licensure test plans
- Certification test plans
- National nursing organization standards
- Accreditation standards and criteria
- State boards of nursing regulations
- Community, practice partners, and stakeholders' input
- Students who are part of the program's stakeholders (Storrar et al., 2019).

The curriculum is revised or developed in a top-down fashion. First, the competency is identified as a knowledge, skill, or attitude the students should possess at the end of the program. Then, the faculty need to identify how that will be accomplished. In other words, competencies are determined as the endpoint or outcome of the curriculum and the process is considered as a means to meet the outcome (Anema & McCoy, 2010). Questions needed to be answered may include:

- At what level should this competency be introduced?
- How will the attainment of this competency be assessed?

2.1 Example Vignette

One standard integrated throughout nursing regulatory and accrediting agencies is evidence-based practice (EBP). At the end of the program, you may expect a baccalaureate nursing student to be able to implement an EBP project and evaluate the project's effectiveness. To reach this competency, the student will have to reach competencies all along the learning process, such as evaluating research literature, developing a researchable question, identifying the data needed to be collected, and analyzing data.

- What content does this competency logically fit with?
- Who is the best facilitator of this competency?
- What is the plan if the benchmark for this competency is not reached by a student?

CURRICULUM FRAMEWORK

Curriculum frameworks organize how students learn cognitive content, psychomotor skills, and affective attributes (or knowledge, skills, and attitude) that are the desired educational outcome of a program (Boland, 2017). Nursing education can use many different types of curriculum organizational schemes, but all frameworks can be congruent with CBE. As the curriculum foundation, competencies can support many different methods of organizing topics.

Traditional and Non-Traditional Frameworks

- Single theory frameworks: one theorist's concepts and assumptions frame nursing content
- Eclectic frameworks: more than one theory organizes the nursing content, for example, Maslow and a nursing theorist
- Non-traditional frameworks: a variety of ideas are used, for example:
  - KSVME Framework—this framework is built around five cornerstones (nursing knowledge, skills, values, meanings, and experience)
  - Healing Web Framework—transformative model around practice that has components of Newman's and Watson's model
  - The Emancipatory Framework—promotes learning through discovery, dialogue, and reflection
  - Quality and Safety Education in Nursing (QSEN) framework, which was developed to promote quality and safety (Boland, 2017).

In addition to the nursing framework, curricula are organized into a schema that can outline course development. Some of the organizations in nursing are:

- Population-based (courses in adult health, psychiatric mental health, maternal-child health)
- Body systems-based (cardiac, respiratory, etc.)
- Concept-based (advocacy, caring, oxygenation, circulation, etc.)

Once nursing faculty decide on a curriculum framework and organization, the competencies can be infused into the system and appropriately placed in courses. In a pure system of CBE, the competencies do not have to be linked to courses.

BOX 2.1   EVIDENCE-BASED TEACHING PRACTICE

The University of Michigan Master of Health Professions Education degree is an example of a fully organized competency-based education. The competencies identified as essential replaced courses, the time frame for competency mastery is flexible and individualized, and the faculty are mentors (University of Michigan, 2019).

THE COPA MODEL

Since 1979, Lenburg has been developing the COPA (Competency Outcomes Performance Assessment) model. The COPA model is composed of four pillars (Figure 2.1).

Lenburg et al. (2009) describe the first pillar as the core practice competencies that include all eight universal competencies (See Table 2.2) integrated in every course and guiding the development of outcome statements.

The essential competencies encompass the major standards of practice for nursing similar to other nursing organizations (Lenburg, 1999). The faculty revising or developing a

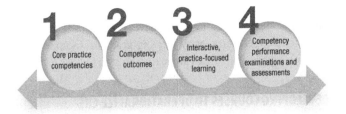

Figure 2.1 The four pillars of the COPA model.

Table 2.2

Eight Universal Core Competencies

Competency	Examples
Assessment and interventions skills	Safety and protection as well as monitoring and treating patients and families
Communication skills	Oral, writing, and computing skills needed to communicate with patients and families, document care, and search for best practice guidelines and evidence
Critical thinking skills	Evaluation of variables and clinical decision-making
Human caring and relationship skills	Legal and ethical considerations as well as cultural humility and patient and family advocacy
Management skills	Prioritization, delegation, and accountability
Leadership skills	Planning, assertiveness, and creativity
Teaching skills	Health promotion and restoration
Knowledge integration skills	Interdisciplinary understanding and interprofessional collaboration

Source: Adapted from Lenburg, C. B. (1999). The framework, concepts, and methods of the competency outcomes and performance assessment (COPA) model. *Online Journal of Issues in Nursing, 4*(3). http://ojin.nursingworld.org/ MainMenuCategories/ANAMarketplace/ANAPeriodicals/

CBE curriculum should look at many different organizational standards and choose one set or develop their own, making sure key competencies every nursing graduate should know for contemporary nursing care are accounted for.

DEVELOPING COURSES TO OPERATIONALIZE CBE

- Course syllabi will outline the competencies for each course and the student learning outcomes or outcome statements. Together, these will map the road more specifically on how to achieve the broader program outcomes or competencies. The learning outcome determines the selection of learning resources.
- Competency writing uses different terms from Bloom et al. (1956) taxonomy compared with student learning outcomes. Competencies are practice-driven, whereas student learning outcomes are content-driven (Anema & McCoy, 2010; Table 2.3).
- The learning resources for each course are aligned with the assessments that evaluate the competencies (Figure 2.2; Johnstone & Soares, 2014).

Table 2.3

Differences in Verbs Used for Competencies and Student Learning Outcomes

Competency Statement	Student Learning Outcomes
Demonstrate a complete physical assessment on an adult.	Describe how to perform a physical assessment of an adult patient.
Integrate two evidence-based best practices when caring for a new mom.	Discuss treatment options with a new mom.
Implement best practice for an oncology patient actively receiving chemotherapy.	List nursing interventions used to reduce the side effects of chemotherapy for an adult.

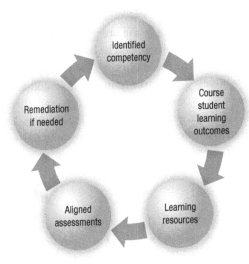

Figure 2.2 Course alignment.

BOX 2.2 EVIDENCE-BASED TEACHING PRACTICE

Due to a lack of orientation processes for new nurse practitioners (NPs), Kopf et al. (2018) developed a competency-based curriculum to assist NP students' transition into practice. Transitioning into practice from academia is stressful, and the authors developed a competency list based on NP practice in the intensive care unit. Competencies were placed in categories that aligned with NP pre-certification education. Competencies were listed under each category and the lists were sent to experts for validation. National experts rated each competency on a Likert scale and nine competency topics were retained.

Once the faculty decides on the program competencies and the framework, the curriculum revision or development can turn to forming syllabi. Course syllabi should reflect CBE by conveying to students the outcome expectations that drive each course and, ultimately, the program competencies. The student learning outcomes should be listed on the syllabi and assist the students in accomplishing the competencies. The students facilitate their learning in all three domains (psychomotor or skills, cognitive or knowledge, and affective or attitude), with each student accomplishing the competencies at a different pace. Benchmarks are set up along the way with no discrete timeline.

Fast Facts

"Competence that is acquired through participation in the program may take place quickly or more slowly, depending on the learner's prior competence level, prior professional activities, motivation, and learning opportunities" (Gruppen et al., 2016).

Some authors describe the benchmarks as "milestones" or concrete behavioral descriptions that are developmental steps to achieve the competency. Competencies encompass multiple domains, which cannot be splintered for assessment in the end (Touchie & Cate, 2016).

Robinson (2018) provides examples of well-defined competencies for the end of an RN-BSN curriculum, which include:

2.2 Example Vignette

If a competency is starting an intravenous infusion on an adult, there is an understanding that communication, professionalism, nursing knowledge, and clinical reasoning skills are integrated into the physical task. The entire patient encounter is assessed as a whole because assessing any one part separately is meaningless when facilitating competency achievement (Touchie & Cate, 2016).

- Make clinical decisions based on the best available evidence
- Prioritize actions based on patient safety needs

Robinson's competencies can then be broken down into course competencies or milestones to be achieved within the curriculum framework. Table 2.4 demonstrates a competency's alignment with a course.

Table 2.4

Alignment of a Competency with Course Student Learning Outcomes

Competency to be met by the End of the Program.	Make clinical decisions based on the best available evidence.		
	Course	Student Learning Outcomes in Courses	Assessment
	Contemporary Nursing Course	Discuss the importance of evidence-based practice in relation to the American healthcare system.	Written paper about process improvement to decrease healthcare errors.
	Nursing Research Course	Categorize evidence according to the Iowa model.	Submit a table of at least five peer-reviewed articles on a clinical topic.
	Nursing Leadership Course	Demonstrate the evidence used to make a clinical decision.	Explain to clinical faculty why a nursing treatment was chosen.

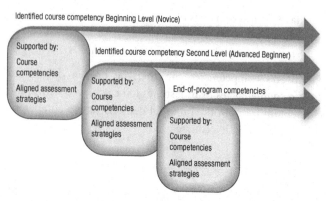

Figure 2.3 CBE course linkages.

Entrustable Professional Activities (EPAs) is a term used in medical schools to map competencies to assessable outcomes or attributes that one would want to see in a healthcare professional.

In CBE, the competency, the content being learned, and the assessment all have a well-defined relationship (Shinners & Graebe, 2019). The course syllabus becomes a concept map for faculty that is leveled within the CBE curriculum. Figure 2.3 connects the pieces making up a CBE course using Benner's (1984) Novice to Expert Theory.

Traditional course development may appear similar to CBE course development, but the difference lies in the outcome. In traditionally graded courses, the students can pass or fail a course but not achieve all the competencies at a satisfactory level. This may occur because the final grade is an average of all course assessments. In CBE, each critical competency needs to be passed at a safe level for the student to move along in the program of study (Anema & McCoy, 2010).

BOX 2.3 EVIDENCE-BASED TEACHING PRACTICE

One method to view competency building has been proposed by Juceviciene and Lepaite (2005), as outlined in Anema and McCoy.

	Type of Competency	Purpose
Level 1	Behavior competencies	To achieve the performance needed in the workplace
Level 2	Added competencies	To improve the work environment using the behavioral competencies with additional knowledge
Level 3	Integrated competencies	To make positive workplace changes using behavioral and added competencies
Level 4	Holistic competencies	To transfer knowledge to new situations

Source: Adapted from Anema, M. G., & McCoy, J. (2010). Competency-based nursing education: A guide to achieving outstanding learning outcomes. Springer Publishing Company (p. 5)

The flexibility of time is one of the most difficult CBE aspects to integrate. Higher education functions on a well-developed time frame, and removing that parameter means revising many academic offices such as Registrar, Financial Aid, Graduation, and Student Services (Gruppen et al., 2016). To "fit in" to an academic schema, many CBE models use the end of the semester as the "outcome point" but leave achievement of milestones flexible within the semester.

ALIGNING EDUCATIONAL ACTIVITIES

Once the syllabi integrate the appropriate leveled competencies that will lead to program competencies or outcomes, faculty have to decide what teaching/learning activities or teaching strategies are relevant for accomplishment of these competencies. In many cases, this means different activities than in traditional educational models because each student needs to practice and achieve a competency in their own time frame. Also, multiple teaching/learning strategies provide flexibility for different types of learners. Some teaching strategies that lend themselves to active learning include:

- Cooperative learning
- Discussions
- Group projects
- Peer tutoring
- Learning cells
- Problem-based learning
- Games
- Simulations
- Portfolios
- Presentations
- Journaling

Fast Facts

"In CBE, the clinical setting becomes an intentional, structured environment for context-specific learning, skill development, and assessment" (Mace & Bacon, 2018, p. 303).

BOX 2.1   EVIDENCE-BASED TEACHING PRACTICE

Mace and Bacon (2018) surveyed athletic trainers ($n = 163$) to find out how much they know about CBE and

(continued)

(continued)

how confident they were in using it as an educational modality. Knowledge and confidence scores were both low, demonstrating that although the term CBE is used in the discipline, faculty needed further information.

LEADERSHIP FOR CURRICULUM REVISION OR DEVELOPMENT

Faculty are the main force propelling a curriculum revision or development, but the task also requires leadership to organize the process. Deciding on a curriculum leader is important, and the curriculum leader needs to understand the content and process of curriculum revision or development (Yoder-Wise, 2013). Curriculum leaders emerge in the following ways:

- *Emergent leadership*—The members of the group view the leader as someone who is knowledgeable and trustworthy; they recognize and accept the leader's influence to lead.
- *Imposed or organizational leadership*—The leader is appointed by someone outside the group. If the group members do not have confidence in the appointed leader's abilities, they may not perform to their highest potential (McHugh, 2017).

Five practices associated with exceptional leadership are as follows:

1. Challenging the process by searching for opportunities, experimenting, and taking risks
2. Inspiring a shared vision by envisioning the future and enlisting the support of others
3. Enabling others to act by fostering collaboration and strengthening others

4. Modeling the way by setting an example and planning small successes
5. Encouraging the heart by recognizing contributions and celebrating accomplishments (Huber, 2000).

Leading curriculum revision or development is challenging because all faculty have invested time and energy into a current curriculum or one they know from previous educational experiences or employment (Venance et al., 2014).

BOX 2.2 EVIDENCE-BASED TEACHING PRACTICE

Venance et al. (2014) used a grounded theory approach to study the perception of faculty ($n = 16$) on curriculum change and what influences faculty engagement. Interviews of faculty about curriculum change revealed three critical change barriers:

1. Tension between individual and institutional values
2. Tension between drivers of change and restrainers of change
3. Tension between perceived gains and perceived losses.

A large driver of change was faculty understanding their part in the change and knowing the rationale for change.

SUMMARY

Revising or developing a curriculum to include CBE takes knowledge, time, and reflection. A strong, visionary leader is needed, as well as faculty who understand the rationale for change and engage in the process. The change begins with reviewing the mission of the organization and educational unit and aligning the change with the needs of the stakeholders. A curriculum framework organizes content and competencies. Milestones are built in to ensure logical succession of competency achievement. Remediation processes are available to ensure success. Assessment and evaluation of competency achievement is completed along the way to ensure student success in reaching program outcomes.

REFERENCES

Anema, M. G., & McCoy, J. (2010). *Competency-based nursing education: A guide to achieving outstanding learning outcomes.* Springer Publishing Company.

Benner, P. (1984). *From novice to expert: Excellence and power in clinical nursing practice.* Addison-Wesley.

Bloom, B. S., Engelhart, M. D., Furst, E. J., Hill, W. H., & Krathwohl, D. R. (1956). *Taxonomy of educational objectives: The classification of educational goals. Handbook I: Cognitive domain.* David McKay Company.

Boland, D. L. (2017). *Developing curriculum: Frameworks, outcomes, and competencies.* Nurse Key. https://nursekey.com/developing-curriculum-frameworks-outcomes-and-competencies/

Ferguson, P. C., Caverzagie, K. J., Nousiainen, M. T., & Snell, L. (2017). Changing the culture of medical training: An important step toward the implementation of competency-based medical education. *Medical Teacher, 39*(6), 599–602. http://dx.doi.org/10.1080/0142159X.2017.1315079

Gruppen, L. D., Burkhardt, J. C., Fitzgerald, J. T., Funnell, M., Haftel, H. M., Lypson, M. L., Mullan, P. B., Santen, S. A., Sheets, K. J., Stalburg, C. M., & Vasquez, J. A. (2016). Competency-based education: Programme design and challenges to implementation. *Medical Education, 50*, 532–539. http://dx.doi.org/10.1111/medu.12977

Huber, D. (2000). *Leadership and nursing care management* (2nd ed.). W. B. Saunders.

Johnstone, S. M., & Soares, L. (2014). Principles for developing competency-based education programs. *Change: The Magazine for Higher Learning, 46*(2), 12–19. https://naspa.tandfonline.com/doi/full/10.1080/00091383.2014.896705#.XQEHlY97nIU

Juceviciene, P., & Lepaite, D. (2005). *Competence as derived from activity: The problem of their level correspondence.* Institute of Educational Studies, University of Technology.

Kopf, R. S., Watts, P. I., Meyer, E. S., & Moss, J. A. (2018). A competency-based curriculum for critical care nurse practitioners' transition to practice. *American Journal of Critical Care, 27*(5), 398–406. http://dx.doi.org/10.4037/ajcc2018101

Lenburg, C. B. (1999). The framework, concepts, and methods of the competency outcomes and performance assessment (COPA) model. *Online Journal of Issues in Nursing, 4*(3). http://ojin.nursingworld.org/MainMenuCategories/ANAMarketplace/ANAPeriodicals/

Lenburg, C. B., Klein, C., Abdur-Rahman, V., Spenser, T., & Boyer, S. (2009). The COPA model: A comprehensive framework designed to promote quality care and competence for patient safety. *Nursing Education Perspectives, 30*(5), 312–317.

Mace, K. L., & Bacon, C. E. W. (2018). Athletic training educators' knowledge and confidence about competency-based education. *Journal of Athletic Training, 13*(4), 302–308. https://doi.org/10.4085/1304302

McHugh, M. L. (2017). Curriculum design and evaluation of program outcomes. In R. Wittmann-Price, M. Godshall, & L. Wilson (Eds.), *Certified Nurse Educator (CNE) review manual.* Springer Publishing Company.

Robinson, F. P. (2018). Competency-based education: An innovative option for nurses. *American Nurse Today, 13*(10), 38–40.

Shinners, J., & Graebe, J. (2019). Continuing professional development: Utilizing competency-based education and the American Nurses Credentialing Center outcome-based continuing education model. *Journal of Continuing Education in Nursing, 50*(3), 100–102. http://dx.doi.org/10.3928/00220124-20190218-02

Storrar, N., Hope, D., & Cameron, H. (2019). Student perspective on outcomes and process: Recommendations for implementing competency-based education. *Medical Teacher, 41*(2), 161–166. http://dx.doi.org/10.3928/00220124-20180517-02

Touchie, C., & Cate, O. (2016). The promise, perils, problems and progress of competency-based medical education. *Medical Education, 50*, 93–100. http://dx.doi.org/10.1111/medu.12839

University of Michigan. (2019). *Master of Health Professions Education.* https://medicine.umich.edu/dept/lhs/education/master-health-professions-education

Venance, S. L., LaDonna, K. A., & Watling, C. J. (2014). Exploring frontline faculty perspectives after a curriculum change. *Medical Education, 48*(10), 998–1007. http://dx.doi.org/10.1111/medu.12529

Yoder-Wise, P. S. (2013). *Leading and managing in nursing* (5th ed.). Elsevier.

3

Implementing Competency-Based Education

Ruth A. Wittmann-Price

"You can't be that kid standing at the top of the water-slide, overthinking it. You have to go down the chute."
— Tina Fey

OBJECTIVES

- Demonstrate methods of writing measurable competencies.
- List the components of the Competency Outcomes and Performance Assessment (COPA) Model.
- Distinguish between a competency statement and an objective.
- Compare different learning and teaching styles.

INTRODUCTION

The implementation of competency-based education (CBE) requires a rethinking of current and traditional educational

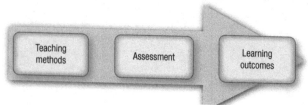

Figure 3.1 Components of CBE.

paradigms. All constituents need to understand the intended learning outcomes to implement CBE. Constituents include:

- Faculty
- Students
- Stakeholders

All the components in CBE have to be aligned to reach the learning outcomes (see Figure 3.1).

KEY IMPLEMENTATION FEATURES

Ideally, students, as stakeholders, should have input into the CBE curriculum. Students, especially, need to understand what is expected of them. Storrar et al. (2019) underscore the importance of providing students with detailed guidance about each competency to complete the learning outcomes. A novice student trying to achieve a competency should understand enough about the "big picture" to understand where and why the competency is needed. Competencies represent two issues for students:

1. Safe clinical practice
2. An assessment

Nursing faculty understand students are worried about assessment and evaluation; therefore, students should know what the assessment entails before evaluation. Faculty mentoring can assist students to prioritize learning needs and apply the competency appropriately into clinical practice. Since many competencies have a psychomotor (skill) component to the cognitive (knowledge) and affective (attitude) domain, only real-world practice opportunities can achieve the competency and integrate the learned skill into the student's professional persona.

Real-world practice has to be clearly defined for students in a CBE model. Faculty supervising students in a clinical situation have to identify if the clinical practice is just "practice" or if it is an evaluative situation (Storrar et al., 2019).

Promoting students' self-determination to achieve competencies promotes professional role development. Storrar et al. (2019) warn against categorizing competencies too distinctly between needed and "extra" because this difference may hamper self-determination. Learners may acquiesce to the minimum standard needed to achieve graduation and not hold themselves to a higher standard to reach competency in the "extras." CBE should promote self-motivation, as achievements build on one another.

COMPETENCY WRITING

To appropriately implement CBE, competency statements must be:

- Realistic
- Leveled
- Understandable
- Measurable

Faculty should understand the difference between developing a competency statement and developing a behavioral learning outcome to implement a CBE model (Table 3.1; Storrar et al., 2019).

COPA MODEL

Lenburg's (1999) COPA (Competency Outcomes and Performance Assessment) model, introduced in Chapter 2, emphasizes the relationship between competency outcomes and appropriate performance assessment (Figure 3.2).

Table 3.1

Comparison of Competency and Behavioral Outcomes	
Competency Outcomes	**Behavioral Outcomes**
Focus on the end result	Focus on content
Reflect the practice environment	May not always reflect practice
Must be in line with current practice	May be traditional and not in line with current practice

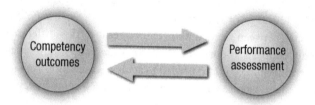

Figure 3.2 COPA model.

The COPA model places competency development and implementation into a framework guided by four questions:

1. What are the essential competencies and outcomes for contemporary practice?
2. What are the indicators that define those competencies?
3. What are the most effective ways to learn those competencies?
4. What are the most effective ways to document that learners and/or practitioners have achieved the required competencies?
   (Lenburg, 1999).

The first question asks faculty to identify essential competencies using current evidence and standards of practice, a key part of the curriculum revision and development. The second question digs down to what indicators need to be placed in the course syllabi to ensure the competencies are defined. The third question dictates the teaching/learning strategies that best promote cognitive (knowledge), psychomotor (skill), and affective (attitude) for competency mastery.

The fourth question challenges nursing faculty to ensure mastery of the competency is validated.

3.1 Example Vignette
An undergraduate student, the clinical nursing instructor, and the acute care hospital are involved in a lawsuit. The student was caring for a patient who had a severe reaction to a medication given to him for the first time by the student. The student noticed the patient's change in status and notified the instructor, the nurse assigned to the patient, and the primary care provider. The family has secured legal counsel about the incident. The attorney requested documentation that the student was competent in giving and monitoring medication administration.
Many nursing programs implement core competencies based on nursing organizations' recommendations as demonstrated in Exhibit 3.1

Exhibit 3.1

Elements of Nursing Organizations Which Can Be Used for Core Competencies in Nursing Education

Nursing Organization	Elements for Core Competencies
American Academy of Colleges of Nursing (AACN, 2008) Essentials of Baccalaureate Education for Professional Nursing Practice	■ Liberal Education ■ Organizational and Systems Leadership ■ Evidence-Based Practice ■ Information Management and Application ■ Health Care Policy ■ Interprofessional Collaboration ■ Population Health ■ Professionalism ■ Patient Care
National League for Nursing (NLN, 2019)	■ Human Flourishing ■ Nursing Judgment ■ Professional Identity ■ Spirit of Inquiry

(continued)

Exhibit 3.1

Elements of Nursing Organizations Which Can Be Used for Core Competencies in Nursing Education (*continued*)

Nursing Organization	Elements for Core Competencies
Quality and Safety Education for Nurses (QSEN, 2019)	<ul><li>Patient Centered Care</li><li>Teamwork and Collaboration</li><li>Evidence-Based Practice</li><li>Quality Improvement</li><li>Safety</li><li>Informatics</li></ul>

Source: American Academy of Colleges of Nursing. (2008). *The essentials of baccalaureate education for professional nursing practice.* http://www.aacnnursing.org/portals/42/publications/baccessentials08 .pdf; National League for Nursing. (2019). *NLN competencies for graduates of nursing programs.* http://www.nln.org/professional-development -programs/competencies-for-nursing-education/nln-competencies-for -graduates-of-nursing-programs; Quality and Safety Education for Nurses. (2019). *QSEN: Quality and safety competencies.* http://qsen.org/ competencies/

The nursing organizations' competency elements have many similarities to each other. In different terms, they all address:

- Safety
- The use of evidence for decision-making
- Leadership
- Quality patient care
- Professionalism

The National League for Nursing (NLN) competencies seem sparse, but they are expanded upon within that model to include core values and integrate concepts that illuminate safety and teamwork (NLN, 2010).

Lenburg (1999) calls the criteria for each competency a subskill to further define "what nurses need to know to be competent graduates." Lenburg discusses core practice competencies and lists them as (1) assessment and intervention, (2) communication, (3) critical thinking, (4) relationship and caring, (5) management, (6) leadership, (7) teaching, and (8) knowledge integration skills.

Lenburg's framework can be used easily by nursing, as can any of the elements identified by the nursing organizations as contemporary competencies needed by graduate nurses. Implementing a system to build up to those competencies requires very measurable outcome statements. Exhibit 3.2 demonstrates a simple nursing example.

Exhibit 3.2

Example of a Competency and Outcomes

Competency: Administer intravenous medication to adult patients.

By the end of this course (session, program, module), the student will be able to:

- Withdraw correct medication and document withdrawal from the system.
- Identify the patient with appropriate patient identifiers.
- Teach the patient about the medication action and side effects.
- Calculate the medication dosage and infusion time.
- Administer the medication using appropriate technique.
- Monitor the patient's response to the medication for 30 minutes.
- Document the administration of the medication according to the standard being used.

In traditional education settings, course objectives may or may not be directly related to practice (Wittmann-Price & Fasolka, 2010). Exhibit 3.3 illustrates an example of these traditional course objectives.

Exhibit 3.3

Example of a Traditional Course Objective

Use safe intravenous medication administration for adult patients.

By the end of this course, the student will be able to:

- Discuss types of medications and their effects on patients.
- Understand the use of intravenous medications as a safe and effective route.
- Differentiate between different antibiotics.
- Describe the process for administering an intravenous medication.

When implementing CBE and developing a competency, the following elements should be considered.

Core Elements of Nursing Competencies

- Student-centered
- Specific
- Concise
- Starts with a verb to describe outcome behavior
- Consistent with nursing standards
- Within the nursing scope of practice
- Part of the abilities needed for a graduate (Lenburg, 1999).

As a nursing faculty group implements CBE curriculum, the preceding attributes can be used as a checklist. Additionally, when developing competencies, Bloom's taxonomy for all three learning domains need to be considered and used from simple to complex to promote student success. Figure 3.3 demonstrates the levels as they move from simple to complex for each domain.

Another aspect or domain of learning important in professional development is "social intelligence." Social intelligence is defined as "the ability to understand others and the **social** context effectively and thus to interact with people successfully" (Yeh, 2013, p. 527). As professionals, it is necessary

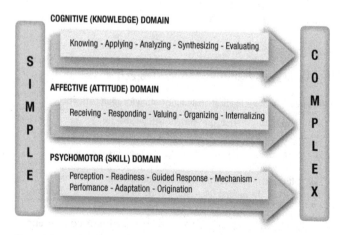

Figure 3.3 Three domains of learning from simple to complex.

BOX 3.1 EVIDENCE-BASED TEACHING PRACTICE

Anderson et al. (2015) studied nurses' literacy, skill, and self-confidence in the competency of applying genomics to health care. To measure the competency, the researchers developed a reliable and valid tool using 16 criteria on a four-point grading scale. Following a review of the literature and use of the tool to evaluate competency, researchers found that knowledge related to up-to-date genome science relevant to nursing practice needed to be developed.

for nursing students to understand and display social intelligence for many reasons, such as:

- Interprofessional collaboration
- Patient and family care and teaching
- Peer support
- Career advancement
- Legal and ethical considerations

Therefore, social intelligence is a component that may need to be evaluated in a CBE model.

BOX 3.2 EVIDENCE-BASED TEACHING PRACTICE

Lee and Woo (2015) studied the relationships among job embeddedness, emotional intelligence (EI), social support, and nursing turnover intention in a statistical model using age, marital status, education, work experience, job title, income, and department as variables ($N = 283$). Results supported the variables of embeddedness, EI, and social support were significantly correlated to turnover intention. EI to turnover intention showed a positive effect. The authors concluded that healthcare organizations should provide EI training and methods for nursing staff to demonstrate their competency.

DELIVERY APPROACHES FOR COMPETENCY-BASED EDUCATION

The method or teaching strategies used to deliver a CBE is dependent on many variables, including:

- Philosophy of the educational organization
- Type of content
- Learning resources available
- Student characteristics
- Faculty ability
- Cost

While face-to-face instruction is the most common delivery, it can be augmented with technology through webcasting, in situ simulation, audience response systems, and computer-assisted modules. Face-to-face can be much more interactive than it once was and provide a rich environment for CBE (Wittmann-Price et al., 2017).

BOX 3.3 EVIDENCE-BASED TEACHING PRACTICE

Terry et al. (2018) completed a quasi-experimental study to compare retention of competence in using an IV infusion pump among **nursing** students ($N = 102$) educated using three different teaching/learning methods (online, face-to-face, and a combination of online and face-to-face). The results of the study supported that **nursing** students retained clinical competence better when **face-to-face** and online learning were combined.

Distance learning usually entails a course platform or a site that contains all the materials needed for a course. Class interactions occur in the discussion area asynchronously or synchronously in a virtual space. Online learning promotes active learning (see Table 3.2).

Table 3.2

Learning Elements in Online Learning	
Facts	Promote review of previous knowledge, such as anatomy and physiology, needed as a foundation for new content
Concepts	Provide ideas and principles needed to make clinical decisions
Procedures	Include step-by-step processes on how to complete a psychomotor competency
Strategies	Know common ways to resolve an issue
Beliefs	Affective knowledge about how personal learning works and includes self-assessment after feedback

Source: Adapted from Farley, M. (2019). The power of perioperative online classrooms. *ORNAC Journal, 37*(2), 13–31.

Nursing faculty take on a different role in CBE than in the traditional teaching style. They become facilitators and motivators. Using teaching styles that build a relationship, providing an interactive learning environment, reminding students when necessary, and guiding them all assists students to achieve competency (Sedden & Clark, 2016).

STUDENT FACTORS

CBE requires a shift in student responsibility. Students must be:

- Self-motivated
- Self-directed
- Able to determine their own pace
- Able to self-reflect
- Able to self-assess (Robinson, 2018).

The learning style of the student is also a factor in CBE. Kolb and Kolb (2005) based their learning style model on four elements or activities that enable students to learn:

1. Sensation
2. Reflex

3. Thinking
4. Doing

From this assumption of four elements and activities, four learning styles were defined and have been validated in studies. The learning styles include:

- Divergent
- Convergent
- Assimilative
- Accommodative

Kolb and Kolb's (2005) learning model integrates the four learning styles to determine where students are in the learning cycle:

- Students who prefer *concrete experimentation* combine the divergent and convergent learning styles and learn through "feeling."
- Students who prefer *reflective observation* combine the convergent and assimilative learning styles and learn through "watching."
- Students who prefer *abstract conceptualization* combine the accommodative and assimilative learning styles and learn through "thinking."
- Students who prefer *active experimentation* combine the divergent and accommodative learning styles and learn through "doing" (Vizeshfar & Torabizadeh, 2018).

Fast Facts

Although no student uses just one learning style, most have a preference. When considering learning styles in relation to CBE, the nursing faculty should incorporate multiple teaching/learning strategies for all students to achieve learning mastery.

SUMMARY

Implementing CBE requires attention to detail in developing the specific competencies for each course. Competency statements need to be measurable and specific so they are achievable and couched in a flexible environment not dependent on time. Benchmarks record achievement. For full implementation of the CBE model, faculty need to consider the learning environment as well as the learning styles of the students. Nursing faculty will enjoy stepping out of their traditional roles and facilitating learning in an interactive environment in which they coach and encourage.

REFERENCES

American Academy of Colleges of Nursing. (2008). *The essentials of baccalaureate education for professional nursing practice.* http://www.aacnnursing.org/portals/42/publications/baccessentials08.pdf

Anderson, G., Alt-White, A. C., Schaa, K. L., Boyd, A. M., & Kasper, C. E. (2015). Genomics for nursing education and practice: Measuring competency. *Worldviews on Evidence-Based Nursing, 12*(3), 165–175. http://dx.doi.org/10.1111/wvn.12096

Farley, M. (2019). The power of perioperative online classrooms. *ORNAC Journal, 37*(2), 13–31.

Kolb, A. E., & Kolb, D. A. (2005). Learning styles and learning spaces: Enhancing experiential learning in higher education. *Academy of Learning and Education, 4*(2), 193–212.

Lee, S., & Woo, H. (2015). Structural relationships among job embeddedness, emotional intelligence, social support and turnover intention of nurses. *Journal of Korean Academy of Nursing Administration, 21*(1), 32–42. http://dx.doi.org/10.11111/jkana.2015.21.1.32

Lenburg, C. B. (1999). The framework, concepts, and methods of the competency outcomes and performance assessment (COPA) model. *Online Journal of Issues in Nursing, 4*(3). http://ojin.nursing world.org/MainMenuCategories/ANAMarketplace/ANA

Periodicals/OJIN/TableofContents/Volume41999/No2Sep1999/COPAModel.html

National League for Nursing. (2010). *Outcome competencies for graduates of practical/vocational, diploma, associate degree, baccalaureate, master's, practice doctorate, and research doctorate programs in nursing.*

National League for Nursing. (2019). *NLN competencies for graduates of nursing programs.* http://www.nln.org/professional-development-programs/competencies-for-nursing-education/nln-competencies-for-graduates-of-nursing-programs

Quality and Safety Education for Nurses. (2019). *QSEN: Quality and safety competencies.* http://qsen.org/competencies/

Robinson, F. P. (2018). Competency-based education: An innovative option for nurses. *American Nurse Today, 13*(10), 38–40.

Sedden, M. L., & Clark, K. R. (2016). Motivating students in the 21st century. *Radiologic Technology, 87*(6), 609–616.

Storrar, N., Hope, D., & Cameron, H. (2019). Student perspective on outcomes ad process: Recommendations for implementing competency-based education. *Medical Teacher, 41*(2), 161–166. http://dx.doi.org/10.3928/00220124-20180517-02

Terry, V. R., Terry, P. C., Moloney, C., & Bowtell, L. (2018). Face-to-face instruction combined with online resources improves retention of clinical skills among undergraduate nursing students. *Nurse Education Today, 61*, 15–19. http://dx.doi.org/10.1016/j.nedt.2017.10.014

Vizeshfar, F., & Torabizadeh, C. (2018). The effect of teaching based on dominant learning style on nursing students' academic achievement. *Nurse Education in Practice, 28*, 103–108. http://dx.doi.org/10.1016/j.nepr.2017.10.013

Wittmann-Price, R. A., & Fasolka, B. (2010). Objectives and outcomes: The fundamental difference. *Nursing Education Perspective, 31*(4), 233–236. http://dx.doi.org/10.1043/1536-5026-31.4.233

Wittmann-Price, M., Godshall, M., & Wilson, L. (2017). *Certified Nurse Educator (CNE) review manual.* Springer Publishing Company.

Yeh, Z. (2013). Role of theory of mind and executive function in explaining social intelligence: A structural equation modeling approach. *Aging and Mental Health, 17*(5), 527–534. http://dx.doi.org/10.1080/13607863.2012.758235

4

Competency-Based Assessments

Karen K. Gittings

"Assessment is today's means of modifying tomorrow's instruction."

— Carol Ann Tomlinson

OBJECTIVES

- Discuss the importance of developing effective assessment tools.
- Identify methods for assessing competency in the cognitive domain.
- Summarize assessment tools that can be used in evaluating the psychomotor domain.
- Explain the challenge in developing methods of assessment for the affective domain.

INTRODUCTION

Developing assessment tools to effectively implement competency-based education (CBE) has progressed over the past couple of decades in many health science disciplines.

Health professional education is experiencing increased accountability from higher education and professional accreditation bodies to produce professionals who are prepared to meet the demands of the complex, fast-paced, ever-changing healthcare environment. Using competency-based assessment methods to evaluate a student's performance can assist in decreasing the gap between education and practice and ease the critical transition from the classroom to the clinic (Henderson, 2016, p. 1).

DEVELOPMENT OF CBE ASSESSMENTS

To develop CBE assessments, tools need to be context specific, reliable, and valid. For example, the Consultation Letter Rating Scale (CLRS) was developed specifically to assess written communication competencies of practitioners (Xu et al., 2019). The evaluation of the CLRS included:

- Validity (was the tool assessing what it was supposed to be assessing?)
- Reliability (was the tool consistent assessment after assessment?)
- Feasibility (was completion of the tool done in a reasonable amount of time?)
- Acceptability (was the tool useful?)

Expert reviewers independently reviewed the CLRS for thematic content and evaluation criteria. Their final reviews showed inter-rater reliability. The process that developed the CLRS shows how to create good assessment tools to determine if competencies (cognitive [knowledge], psychomotor [skills], and affective [attitude]) are met in future nurses and healthcare professionals.

Fast Facts

There are three different types of validity.

- Content validity—does the assessment tool align with the competency?
- Face validity—does the assessment measure what it actually intends to measure?
- Construct validity—do the test or assessment items perform as intended to measure the content? (Begley et al., 2018).

Henderson (2016) developed an assessment tool for occupational therapy students to measure clinical performance competencies. Development started with a review of professional literature.

Knowing what to assess is the beginning point. First, know what competencies are needed to function effectively and safely as a professional nurse, and afterward identify the assessment constructs. Expert advice on what competencies are needed by graduating nurses can be gleaned in a multitude of ways, such as a thorough literature review, through structured observation of current practice, and/or quality improvement processes.

COMPETENCY DOMAINS

Next, decide on the domains of the competency. Domains can be outlined by regulatory or accreditation organizational standards (Henderson, 2016) and matrixed with learning domains. For example, the National Council of State Boards of Nursing (NCSBN) uses a high-stakes assessment to determine minimal competency for nursing licensure. The licensure examination for registered professional nurses has the practice broken into eight domains that include:

- Management of care
- Safety and infection control

- Health promotion and maintenance
- Psychosocial integrity
- Basic care and comfort
- Pharmacological and parenteral therapies
- Reduction of risk potential
- Physiological adaptation (NCSBN, 2019).

To determine competency, studies are ongoing about what graduate nurses actually do, think, and learn in clinical settings. Competency is difficult to define. Not every nurse or healthcare professional demonstrates competency to the same degree or in every situation (NCSBN, 2014).

BOX 4.1 EVIDENCE-BASED TEACHING PRACTICE

Jensen et al. (2018) used the Delphi Method with an international group of experts to develop a tool to assess very specific surgical competencies. After four rounds of questionnaires, experts reached consensus in eight different competency categories. The assessment tool has been used successfully and consistently.

4.1 Example Vignette

When developing a CBE assessment for occupational therapy students, Henderson (2016) used six domains:

- *Communication*
- *Documentation*
- *Safety and judgment*
- *Evaluation*
- *Intervention*
- *Professional behaviors.*

BOX 4.2 EVIDENCE-BASED TEACHING PRACTICE

Melvin and Cavalcantie (2016) used case presentations with medical students to assess competencies in three separate domains: data gathering, clinical reasoning, and verbal presentation. To use the case presentation assessment to assess competencies, the following expectations were put in place, including: developing clear goals for the tutor and learner, using probing or Socratic questions to assess the presenter's knowledge, and providing specific feedback to each learner.

Fast Facts

There are three learning domains:

1. Cognitive (Knowledge)
2. Psychomotor (Skill)
3. Affective (Attitude)

Students' cognitive or knowledge development builds from simple to complex. The cognitive pinnacle for nursing students is good clinical decision-making based on best evidence, patient preference, and ethical consideration within the professional nurse's scope of practice.

Cognitive assessment is usually founded on Bloom's (1956) taxonomy for educational objectives. Although Bloom intended the taxonomy to span cognitive, psychomotor, and affective domains, the taxonomy is used most often for cognitive assessment purposes. Bloom's domains span from simple (remembering) to complex (creating), as demonstrated in Figure 4.1.

Assessment items can be both qualitative and statistical. They can include test items, Likert scale items, continuums,

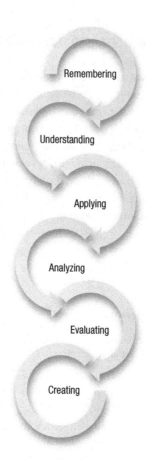

Figure 4.1 Bloom's taxonomy in figure format.

multiple-choice questions (MCQ), multiple multiples questions, demonstration, observation, etc. Once the appropriate type of item is matched with the construct being measured, it should be beta tested or pilot tested (Bustraan et al., 2016). Additionally, some competencies, especially end-of-program competencies, can be assessed using technological methods, such as computerized adaptive testing (CAT; Petersen et al., 2016).

COGNITIVE COMPETENCIES

The knowledge domain competencies are often assessed using test items. Once the faculty have defined the cognitive domains requiring assessment, they will need items to elicit those domains at the correct cognitive level. The recognition of Item Response Theory (IRT), also known as the latent response theory, can help choose assessment items. IRT is a measurement model that considers:

- The human variables of assessment
- The item parameters of the assessment
- The mathematical functions of the human and item parameters
  (Thomas, 2019).

The IRT model considers unobservable elements such as personality traits, which can include stress and anxiety, as well as knowledge (Columbia University, Mailman School of Public Health, 2019). A graphic depiction on IRT is demonstrated in Figure 4.2

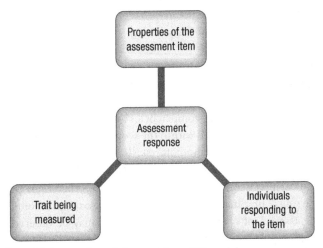

Figure 4.2 Interaction of elements in an IRT model.

BOX 4.3 EVIDENCE-BASED TEACHING PRACTICE

Trakman et al. (2017) developed a CBE assessment tool using an eight-step process:

1. Define the construct and develop a test plan.
2. Develop the test items.
3. Choose the scoring system and format.
4. Assess the content validity.
5. Assess the face validity.
6. Perform test item analysis (difficulty and discrimination).
7. Evaluate reliability of scale.
8. Assess construct validity.

BOX 4.4 EVIDENCE-BASED TEACHING PRACTICE

Raymond et al. (2019) studied MCQ used for assessment and found that almost half of all test items ($n = 840$) had one to two non-functional distractors, thereby increasing the chance of correct guessing.

PSYCHOMOTOR COMPETENCY ASSESSMENT

Many times, "nursing competencies" refers to psychomotor demonstration of a skill within the scope and practice of professional nursing. Psychomotor skills are most often evaluated within the skills or simulation laboratories and/or the clinical practicum area. Frequently, people other than the nursing course instructor may have input into the psychomotor assessment of the student; the student may be observed by part-time faculty, as well as patients and families. Due to accreditation and academic criteria, the nursing faculty usually provides the summative (course) grade.

Psychomotor competency-based assessments can be developed with a pass/fail scale (dichotomous-based) or a graded/rated scale. On a graded/rated scale, the nursing faculty need to agree on the minimum level of acceptable competency and use this level consistently. Graded/rated scales are criterion-based once a needed competency is identified. After the faculty identify the competency, they must set a goal or acceptable level of achievement. Graded/rated levels of psychomotor competencies are usually predicated on rubrics providing quantifiable assessments for each grade or rating. Rubrics further explain the criteria for an acceptable grade/rating compared to an unacceptable or an exceptional grade/rating. The Bondy (1983) scale is a widely used five-point rating assessment. (Table 4.1).

The Bondy Scale has a 0 to 5 scoring system. Each score has a label, and the criteria to apply the score is explained by describing the standard of procedure, the quality of the performance expected, and the level of assistance or supervision required. By qualifying each criterion, the assessment scale is easier to use and provides clearer feedback to students, which should promote reflection on their psychomotor performance.

AFFECTIVE COMPETENCY ASSESSMENT

Professionalism and other nursing values held in high esteem, like advocacy, integrity, and caring, are the most difficult to assess and are interrelated with cognitive and psychomotor assessments.

Fast Facts

Nursing organizations have promoted renewing nursing's professional identity in students as one important element of promoting patient safety and retention of nursing staff (Schmidt & McArthur, 2018).

Table 4.1

The Bondy (1983) Scale for Nursing Skill Assessment

Scale Label	Score	Standard of Procedure	Quality of Performance	Level of Assistance Required
Independent	5	Safe Accurate Achieved intended outcome Behavior is appropriate to context	Proficient Confident Expedient	No supporting cues required
Supervised	4	Safe Accurate Achieved intended outcome Behavior is appropriate to context	Proficient Confident Reasonably expedient	Requires occasional supportive cues
Assisted	3	Safe Accurate Achieved most objectives for intended outcome Behavior generally appropriate to context	Proficient throughout most of performance when assisted	Required frequent verbal and occasional physical directives in addition to supportive cues

Marginal	2	Safe only with guidance Not completely accurate Incomplete achievement of intended outcome	Unskilled Inefficient	Required continuous verbal and frequent physical directive cues
Dependent	1	Unsafe Unable to demonstrate behavior Lack of insight into behavior appropriate to context	Unskilled Unable to demonstrate behavior/procedure	Required continuous verbal and continuous physical directive cues
X	0	Not Observed		

Source: Copyright permissions were granted.

Professional Identity in nursing is defined as "a sense of one-self, and in relationship with others, that is influenced by the characteristics, norms and values of the nursing discipline, resulting in the individual thinking, acting and feeling like a nurse" (Godfrey & Crigger, 2017, p. 379). Professionalism and all associated attributes are correlated with self-efficacy and the actual "calling" to be a nurse (Hyewon & Sujeong, 2019).

BOX 4.5 EVIDENCE-BASED TEACHING PRACTICE

Aydin et al. (2017) surveyed first- and fourth-year nursing students (*N* = 120) to identify their perceptions of professionalism. They found first-year students most frequently identified "professional competence" as the leading element of professionalism. The fourth-year students most often identified "responsibility." Other attributes of professionalism identified by first-year students were "geniality," "patience," "calmness," "love of nursing," "loyalty to nursing," and "not attaching importance to material values." Other attributes identified by fourth-year students were "empathy," "honesty," "responsibility," and "scientific curiosity." The study demonstrated how the perception of professionalism grew over time with knowledge and skill development.

Affective or attitude competencies are often intermixed and assessed with knowledge and psychomotor competencies. It is difficult to isolate knowledge and psychomotor from affective assessment. How a student approaches learning or a clinical decision is as important as knowing why they are doing something and implementing the task correctly. Many nursing programs know how to provide a negative assessment

Exhibit 4.1

Affective Competency Assessment Example

LEARNING OUTCOME #8

	X	1	2	3	4	5	Comment
8. Demonstrates professionalism and the inherent values of altruism, autonomy, human dignity, integrity, and social justice, which are fundamental to the discipline of nursing.							
a. Applies principles of legal core values of nursing and social justice in the delivery of patient care.							
b. Discusses ethical issues involved with patient care and their implications on the patient, family, and society.							
c. Behaves professionally and abides by nursing's student policies as listed in the Student Handbook.							
d. Arrives to the clinical site in a timely manner to provide consistent patient care and dresses in professional attire for the clinical day.							
e. Utilizes constructive criticism and changes behavior accordingly.							
f. Abides by the ANA Code of Ethics and established guidelines of the SC Nurse Practice Act.							

list or can identify "lack of professionalism," but quantifying attributes such as calmness and empathy are much more subjective. Additionally, there may not be opportunities to observe affective attributes such as patient advocacy, unless advocacy is broadly defined by faculty. Since many affective competency-based assessments are intermingled with clinical skill assessment in the actual patient area, they sometimes fall within the psychomotor assessment tool. An example of an affective assessment is demonstrated in a clinical assessment tool in Exhibit 4.1.

The affective competencies above are based on the American Association of Colleges of Nursing's (AACN) *The Essentials of Baccalaureate Education for Professional Nursing Practice* (2008) number VIII essential, which states "Professionalism and the inherent values of altruism, autonomy, human dignity, integrity, and social justice are fundamental to the discipline of nursing" (p. 4). The scale in the above competencies is based on the Bondy Scale (1984).

SUMMARY

Competency-based assessment methods can decrease the gap from education to practice. To be effective, they must be specific, reliable, and valid. Domains of competency may be prescribed by the regulatory or accrediting bodies for professional programs, but learning is traditionally categorized into the three domains of cognitive (knowledge), psychomotor (skill), and affective (attitude). Competency within the cognitive domain is often assessed through testing. Psychomotor competencies are usually assessed in the skills/simulation laboratories and/or practicum areas. Affective competencies are more difficult to assess, so they are often done in conjunction with an assessment of cognitive or psychomotor competency. CBE requires the development of assessment methods that are effective in evaluating competency in the three traditional domains of learning.

REFERENCES

American Association of Colleges of Nursing. (2008). *The essentials of baccalaureate education for professional nursing practice.* http://www.aacnnursing.org/portals/42/publications/bacces sentials08.pdf

Aydin, E. R., Mine, M., & Akpinar, A. (2017). Attributes of a good nurse: The opinions of nursing students. *Nursing Ethics, 24*(2), 238–248. http://dx.doi.org.fmarion.idm.oclc.org/10.1177/09697 33015595543

Begley, A., Paynter, E., & Dhaliwal, S. S. (2018). Evaluation tool development for food literacy programs. *Nutrients, 10*(11), 1617. http://dx.doi.org/10.3390/nu10111617

Bloom, B. S. (1956). *Taxonomy of educational objectives: The classification of educational goals.* Addison-Wesley Longman.

Bondy, K. N. (1983). Criterion-referenced definitions for rating scales in clinical evaluation. *Journal of Nursing Education, 22*(9), 376–382.

Bustraan, J., Henry, W., Kortbeek, J. B., Brasel, K. J., Hofmann, M., & Schipper, I. B. (2016). MCQ tests in advanced trauma life support (ATLS): Development and revision. *Injury, 47*(3), 665–668. http://dx.doi.org/10.1016/j.injury.2015.11.024

Columbia University, Mailman School of Public Health. (2019). *Item response theory.* https://www.mailman.columbia.edu/research/population-health-methods/item-response-theory

Godfrey, N., & Crigger, N. (2017). Professional identity. In J. Giddens (Ed.), *Concepts of nursing practice* (2nd ed.). Elsevier.

Henderson, W. (2016). Development of a clinical performance assessment tool for an occupational therapy teaching clinical. *Open Journal of Occupational Therapy, 4*(3), 1–14. http://dx.doi.org/10.15453/2168-6408.1217

Hyewon, K., & Sujeong, H. (2019). Mediating effects of self-efficacy between calling and nursing professionalism for nurses in general hospitals. *Journal of Korean Academy of Nursing Administration, 25*(3), 220–228. http://dx.doi.org.fmarion.idm.oclc.org/10.11111/jkana.2019.25.3.220

Jensen, K., Petersen, R. H., Hansen, H. J., Walker, W., Pedersen, J. H., & Knoge, L. (2018). A novel assessment tool for evaluating competence in video-assisted thoracoscopic surgery lobectomy.

Surgical Endoscopy, 32(10), 4173–4182. http://dx.doi.org/10.1007/ s00464018-6162-8

Melvin, L., & Cavalcantie, R. B. (2016). The oral case presentation: A key tool for assessment and teaching in competency-based medical education. *JAMA, 316*(21), 2187–2188. http://dx.doi .org/10.1001/jama.2016.16415

National Council of State Boards of Nursing. (2014). *How competent are we in assessing competency?* https://www.ncsbn.org/ IRE_2014_ZAustin.pdf

National Council State Boards of Nursing. (2019). *NCLEX-RN® examination test plan for the National Council Licensure Examination for Registered Nurses.* https://www.ncsbn.org/2019_RN _TestPlan-English.pdf

Petersen, M., Aaronson, N., Chie, W., Conroy, T., Costantini, A., Hammerlid, E., Hjermstad, M., Kaasa, S., Loge, J., Velikova, G., Young, T., & Groenvold, M. (2016). Development of an item bank for computerized adaptive test (CAT) measurement of pain. *Quality of Life, 25*(1), 1–11. http://dx.doi.org/10.1007/ s11136-015-1069-5

Raymond, M. R., Stevens, C., & Bucak, S. D. (2019). The optimal number of options for multiple-choice questions on high-stakes tests: Application of a revised index for detecting nonfunctional distractors. *Advances in Health Sciences Education, 24*(1), 141–150. http://dx.doi.org/10.1007/s10459-018-9855-9

Schmidt, B. J., & McArthur, E. C. (2018). Professional nursing values: A concept analysis. *Nursing Forum, 53*(1), 69–75. http:// dx.doi.org/10.1111/nuf.12211

Thomas, M. L. (2019). Advances in applications of item response theory to clinical assessment. *Psychological Assessment, 31*(12), 1442–1455. http://dx.doi.org/10.1037/pas0000597

Trakman, G. L., Forsyth, A., Hoye, R., & Belski, R. (2017). Developing and validating a nutrition knowledge questionnaire: Key methods and considerations. *Public Health Nutrition, 20*(15), 2670–2679. http://dx.di.org/10.1017/S1368980017001471

Xu, V. Y. Y., Hamid, J., von Maltzahn, M., Izukawa, T., Norris, M., Chau, V., Liu, B., & Wong, C. (2019). Use of the Consultant Letter Rating Scale among geriatric medicine postgraduate trainees. *Journal of the American Geriatric Society, 67*(10), 2157–2160. http://dx.doi.org/10.111/jgs.1

5

Evaluating Competencies

Rev. Robert G. Mulligan

"You may explore; you may evaluate but you can't exe-cute if you are not willing to take action. Decide to take off now!"

—Israelmore Ayivor

OBJECTIVES

- Demonstrate understanding of the concepts of assessment and evaluation.
- Explain and give examples of cognitive, affective, and psychomotor competency evaluation.
- Understand and explain the concept of evidence-based teaching practice and evidence-based evaluation.
- Explain how the use of rubrics and scales can contribute to evidence-based evaluation.

INTRODUCTION

Assessment Versus Evaluation

Educators often confuse assessment and evaluation, thinking them interchangeable. An assessment is any means of obtaining information to measure an outcome. The main purpose of an assessment is to understand and improve student learning. An assessment is a formative evaluation, a process to determine progress with the goal of making improvements. Evaluation is more commonly associated with summative evaluation. A summative evaluation judges the value and quality of performance in the final stage of observation. In the clinical setting, the summative evaluation is the point of decision in candidate performance. Faculty in clinical disciplines must evaluate student attainment of course outcomes and defined program competencies.

Evaluating competency is more than evaluating knowledge; it also evaluates the application of knowledge in real-world situations. Evaluating knowledge, skills, and affective behavior all starts with competencies based on sound standards that are criterion referenced. The criteria developed from sound standards should be tested in an environment that is an equal playing field for all students. Evaluations gather evidence to substantiate a student has reached a set competency.

Additionally, individual student evaluations of competency are data for evaluating program outcomes. Program outcomes assessment or evaluation is developed long before individual data is collected. Program outcomes should, of course, be related to the mission of the program and benchmarked. Program outcome data is needed for recognizing achievements and ongoing process improvement.

> ### 5.1 Example Vignette
>
> *A nursing program outcome is one-year alumni satisfaction with the program on an average of 4.0 on a 1 to 5 Likert scale. The current survey has a 17% return rate and overall satisfaction of 3.89. The process improvement process included:*
>
> 1. *Reviewing capacity building among nursing faculty for student interaction*
> 2. *An approach to analyze student perceptions of the program*
> 3. *In-depth content review of student schedules and expectations*
> 4. *Follow-up and monitoring*
>
> *Identification for areas of process improvement were then subject to Plan, Do, Study, Act (PDSA) plans to make effective and enduring changes, as well as to reevaluate changes as they are made (Farrell & Clarkin, 2020).*

DEVELOPMENT OF CBE EVALUATIONS

Evaluative mechanisms to "judge" or determine a competency has been met should be varied because learners have varied learning styles. Much of competency-based education (CBE) is related to psychomotor behavior because it is observable. Competencies for nurses and all healthcare professionals must be met in all three learning domains to verify graduating students are well-rounded, safe practitioners.

Evaluators must recognize all learning domains are interrelated. Students do not provide safe care without knowledge (cognitive) about why they are implementing a procedure (psychomotor) while providing the patient and family with a psychologically safe environment (affective).

Griffiths et al. (2019) studied CBE evaluation thorough a qualitative grounded study. They found the CBE was spurring new evaluation processes within healthcare programs. Three themes extracted from the research interviews include:

1. Specific identified shifts in assessment culture
2. Factors supporting the shifts in culture
3. Outcomes related to the culture shift

Overall, the researchers found internal and external support for CBE evaluations for students and programs.

Placing competencies into domains assists nursing faculty in developing appropriate evaluation mechanisms. Competencies are often organized into domains, or categories of learning outcomes, as defined by Bloom's taxonomy of learning domains. Horrocks et al. (2019) used the method successfully for disaster response education. The competencies were divided into core competencies and specialized competencies for evaluation purposes.

Competency evaluation can, and many times should, be interprofessional. Lewis et al. (2019) looked at the evaluations of clinical performance of direct patient care across healthcare disciplines. Participants ($N = 2,223$) included nurses and midwives who scored the highest, associate clinicians, and physicians. The results indicated substantial gaps in clinical performance among recently graduated practitioners, raising concerns about the traditional educational model. The study also indicated there are necessary competencies for all health professionals to attain.

COGNITIVE COMPETENCY EVALUATION

The cognitive domain involves knowledge and the development of intellectual skills (Bloom, 1956). This includes the recall or recognition of specific facts, procedural patterns, and concepts that serve in the development of intellectual abilities and skills. There are six major categories in the cognitive domain, from the simplest to the most complex:

- Knowledge
- Comprehension
- Application
- Analysis
- Synthesis
- Evaluation

Anderson et al. (2000) revisited Bloom's cognitive domain in the mid-nineties, which resulted in the renaming of the categories. Table 5.1 provides a summary of these categories.

Multiple methods can verify students' acquisition of knowledge. Some nursing programs, such as Roseman University of Health Sciences (RUHS), designed their entire program on "mastery learning" or CBE. Although there is little outcome data for CBE nursing programs, RUHS defined competency achievement as ≥90% on an assessment. The RUHS program increased program outcomes, including:

- National licensure scores
- Student satisfaction
- Student retention

RUHS demonstrated that CBE can produce competent entry-level nurses (Linsky et al., 2019).

Table 5.1

Cognitive Competency Categories	
Remembering	Recalling information
Understanding	Comprehending information; interpreting instructions
Applying	Using information in a new situation
Analyzing	Understanding component parts and organizing them
Evaluating	Making a value judgment
Creating	Building something new from diverse elements

BOX 5.1 EVIDENCE-BASED TEACHING PRACTICE

The Association for Gerontology in Higher Education (AGHE) has adopted competencies needed in the curriculum for both undergraduate and graduate healthcare professionals. Dassel et al. (2019) used curriculum mapping to align competencies with measurable objectives and relate the appropriate evaluation mechanism to the competency.

BOX 5.2 EVIDENCE-BASED TEACHING PRACTICE

Researchers Dunne et al. (2020) identified 12 "Entrustable Professional Activities (EPA)," which could be labeled as competencies needed for practitioners caring for people with HIV. The EPAs were used to guide the curriculum development and teaching/learning activities of an Internal Residency program. Evaluation tools based on the EPAs were also developed for use in the program. The evaluations demonstrated that graduates were ready for unsupervised practice in 91% of EPAs at the end of the 3-year program.

PSYCHOMOTOR COMPETENCY EVALUATION

The psychomotor domain (Simpson, 1972) includes physical movement, coordination, and use of the motor-skill areas. They range from manual tasks, such as digging a ditch or washing a car, to more complex tasks, such as operating a complex piece of machinery or dancing. Development of these skills requires practice and is measured in terms of speed, precision, distance, procedures, or techniques in execution. Table 5.2 lists the seven major categories from the simplest behavior to the most complex.

Table 5.2

Psychomotor Competency Categories	
Perception	Attending to sensory clues
Set	Mental, physical, emotional disposition
Guided Response	Learning by imitation
Mechanism	Learning a complex skill; achieving proficiency
Complex Overt Response	Quick and coordinated performance of motor skills
Adaptation	The ability to modify motor skills
Origination	The ability to develop new movements for a particular situation

BOX 5.3 EVIDENCE-BASED TEACHING PRACTICE

Desai et al. (2018) reviewed competency-based assessments for interventional pulmonology (IP) and found several well-validated tools to measure most commonly performed procedures, but other procedures lacked evaluative assessments. The researchers also found that using simulation experiences to practice procedures increased positive outcomes in students.

AFFECTIVE COMPETENCY EVALUATION

The affective domain (Krathwohl et al., 1973) includes how we deal with things emotionally, such as feelings, *values*, appreciation, enthusiasm, motivation, and *attitudes*. Table 5.3 lists the five major categories from the simplest behavior to the most complex.

Table 5.3

Affective Competency Categories	
Receiving	Awareness, willingness to hear, selected attention
Responding	Active participation on the part of the learners; attend to and react to
Valuing	Internalization of values as seen in changed behavior
Organization	Organizing and prioritizing values; resolving conflicts between values
Internalizing	Internalizing values; value system controls behavior

Assessing affective competencies in students may be one of the more difficult evaluations. Attributes like advocacy and professionalism need clear definition by the faculty performing the evaluations. Many evaluation tools for affective competency are based on negatives rather than positive behavior; nursing faculty are more likely to identify what is not "professionalism" than what demonstrates professionalism.

To develop affective and interpersonal skills among healthcare providers, health professions' education programs must build student competencies in the affective domain of learning. Donlan (2018) investigated strategies used to evaluate affective domain learning in health professions' education, including:

- The think-pair-share technique
- Reflective journaling
- Simulation and role play
- Motivational interviewing
- Structured controversy

Additionally, Donlan found technology-based learning platforms can either facilitate or produce barriers to affective learning. Also important in affective learning are:

- Faculty approach
- Student feedback
- Course design

Donlan suggests affective learning competencies are best achieved when teaching practices emphasize:

- Self-awareness
- Multiple points of view
- Perspective transformation
- Interpersonal skills
- Person-centered care

BOX 5.4 EVIDENCE-BASED TEACHING PRACTICE

Evans et al. (2017) developed an electronic evaluation tool from a Humanitarian Competency Framework. Using simulation as a method, the evaluation tool was used formatively and summatively to assess five global competencies. Additionally, all participants used the tool to self- and peer-evaluate. The results demonstrated that self-evaluation scores were lower than peer-evaluation scores and participants with a healthcare background or prior humanitarian work scored higher. The tool is being tested for general use to assess humanitarian competencies.

PROVIDING EFFECTIVE FEEDBACK IN EVALUATION

Marzano et al. (2018) states effective feedback begins with clearly defined and clearly communicated learning goals. Proficiency scales and rubrics allow students to know their level of knowledge and if they have achieved the appropriate program benchmark. A rubric is tied to a particular

Table 5.4

Rubric and Scale to evaluate Cognitive, Affective, and Psychomotor Competencies

Domain	Unsatisfactory 0	Satisfactory 1	Emerging 2	Proficient 3	Outstanding 4
Cognitive					
Licensure exam scores					
Completion of benchmarks in curriculum mapping					
Psychomotor					
Use of tools to measure commonly performed procedures					
Affective					
Interpersonal skills					
Advocacy					
Self-awareness					
Professionalism					
Total	0	3	6	9	12

Formative Evaluation: A candidate must achieve a total score of at least "3" with no score of "0" in any category. The evaluator will make suggestions for improvement.

Summative Evaluation: A candidate must achieve a score of at least "9" with no score below "3" to advance in the program.

domain or task. A scale describes the progression in knowledge and understanding of that domain or task (Marzano et al., 2018).

Rubrics and scales allow for candidate self-evaluation and can serve as a tool for metacognition. By allowing for greater reliability and validity in evaluation of a candidate, they can increase inter-observer reliability if used by teams (Moskal, 2000). For an example rubric and scale, see Table 5.4.

Whenever possible, rubrics and scales should be shared with the students in advance to allow students the opportunity to provide evidence that they have met the criteria (Moskal, 2000).

SUMMARY

Evaluation, which usually occurs at the end of a performance and is referred to as summative, is often confused with assessment, which involves obtaining additional information for decision-making. In evaluating students, evaluate not only knowledge attainment, but also knowledge application. It is essential to evaluate nursing students for competency in preparation for their transition to practice. Competency should be evaluated in the three domains: cognitive, psychomotor, and affective. Along with evaluation of competency, feedback provides additional information for improvement and future learning.

REFERENCES

Anderson, L. W., Krathwohl, D. R., Airasian, P. W., Cruikshank, K. A., Mayer, R. E., Pintrich, P. R., Raths, J., & Wittrock, M. C. (2001). *A taxonomy for learning, teaching, and assessing: A revision of Bloom's taxonomy of educational objectives.* Pearson, Allyn & Bacon.

Bloom, B. S. (Ed.). (1956). *Taxonomy of educational objectives: The classification of educational goals. Handbook I: Cognitive domain.* Longmans, Green & Co. Ltd.

Dassel, K., Eaton, J., & Felsted, K. (2019). Navigating the future of gerontology education curriculum mapping to the AGHE competencies. *Gerontology and Geriatrics Education, 40*(1), 132–138. http://dx.doi.org/10.1080/02701960.2018.1500908

Desai, N. R., Parikh, M. S., & Lee, H. J. (2018). Interventional pulmonology: The role of simulation training and competency-based evaluation. *Seminars in Respiratory and Critical Care Medicine, 39*(6), 747–754. http://dx.doi.org/10.1055/s-0038-1677469

Donlan, P. (2018). Developing affective domain learning in health professions education. *Journal of Allied Health, 47*(4), 289–295.

Dunne, D., Green, M., Tetrault, J., & Barakat, L. A. (2020). Development of a novel competency-based evaluation system for HIV primary care training: The HIV entrustable professional activities. *JGIM: Journal of General Internal Medicine, 35*(1), 331–335. http://dx.doi.org/10.1007/s11606-019-04956-1

Evans, A. B., Hulme, J. M., Nugus, P., Cranmer, H. H., Coutu, M., & Johnson, K. (2017). An electronic competency-based evaluation tool for assessing humanitarian competencies in a simulated exercise. *Prehospital and Disaster Medicine, 32*(3), 253–260. http://dx.doi.org/10.1017/S1049023X1700005X

Farrell, B., & Clarkin, C. (2020). Community pharmacists as catalysts for deprescribing: An exploratory study using quality improvement processes. *Canadian Pharmacists Journal, 153*(1), 37–45. http://dx.doi.org.proxy1.lib.tju.edu/10.1177/1715163519882969

Griffiths, J., Dalgarno, N., Schultz, K., Han, H., & van Melle, E. (2019). Competency-based medical education implementation: Are we transforming the culture of assessment? *Medical Teacher, 41*(7), 811–818. http://dx.doi.org/10.1080/0142159X.2019.1584276

Horrocks, P., Hobbs, L., Tippett, V., & Aitken, P. (2019). Paramedic disaster health management competencies: A scoping review.

Prehospital and Disaster Medicine, 34(3), 322–329. https://doi.org/10.1017/S1049023X19004357

Krathwohl, D. R., Bloom, B. S., & Masia, B. B. (1973). *Taxonomy of educational objectives: The classification of educational goals. Handbook II: Affective domain.* David McKay Co.

Lewis, T. P., Roder-DeWan, S., Malata, A., Ndiave, Y., & Kruk, M. E. (2019). Clinical performance among recent graduates in nine low- and middle-income countries. *Tropical Medicine and International Health, 24*(5), 620–635. https://doi.org/10.1111/tmi.13224

Linsky, M. S., Cone, C. J., Watson, S., Lawrence, P. T., & Lutfivva, M. N. (2019). Mastery learning in a bachelor's of nursing program: The Roseman University of Health Sciences experience. *BMC Nursing, 18*(1), 52. https://doi.org/10.1186/s12912-019-0371-x

Marzano, R., Norford, J. S., & Ruyle, M. (2018). The new art and science of classroom assessment. *Solution Tree.* https://www.solutiontree.com/new-art-and-science-of-classroom-assessment.html

Moskal, B. M. (2000). Scoring rubrics: What, when and how? *Practical Assessment, Research, and Evaluation, 7*(3). https://doi.org/10.7275/a5vq-7q66

Simpson, E. J. (1972). *The classification of educational objectives in the psychomotor domain.* Gryphon House.

6

Educational Process Improvement

Evelyn (Evie) Lengetti

"As indispensable members of the healthcare team, nurses today are at the forefront of advancing evidence-based solutions and leading innovation in an atmosphere of accelerating change."

—AACN

OBJECTIVES

- Describe a framework for educational process improvement.
- Apply this framework to the practice of teaching from a macro and micro perspective.

INTRODUCTION

Education Process Improvement (EPI) can be described by borrowing and applying the works of both Avedis Donabedian, MD, and W. Edwards Deming. The Donabedian framework provides a macro perspective for EPI. This macro perspective reflects the systems and structures set forth by the school or college of nursing. For a different view, Deming's quality improvement cycle guides the teaching strategies used to instruct students. This micro perspective shows the process for instruction and feedback that is evidence-based and individualized to the student's performance. EPI assists curricula to move from a traditional pedagogy to competency-based education methods.

EDUCATIONAL PROCESS IMPROVEMENT

Macro View: Donabedian EPI Framework

To align the Donabedian framework with a nursing program, *structure* means the formal administrative support that ensures faculty have access to the most current information, the right tools to deliver the education, and the right place to conduct the education, such as in a simulation center or a patient's bedside. Structure can also refer to professional external agencies such as the American Association of Colleges of Nursing (AACN). *Process* describes how the program makes all faculty aware of external standards of care, assures adherence and application of the AACN Essentials in practice, and confirms all faculty are current with and practicing evidence-based standards of care. *Outcomes* are true measures of students' success and can also be determinants of future performance (Ayanian & Markel, 2016). As educators, you cannot separate the structure, process, and outcome when evaluating competence. Donabedian's Model for quality assessment provides a framework for EPI (Figure 6.1).

Fast Facts

"Given the growing body of evidence linking education to quality outcomes, employers increasingly expect registered nurses to be prepared at the baccalaureate level" (AACN, 2019, p. 3).

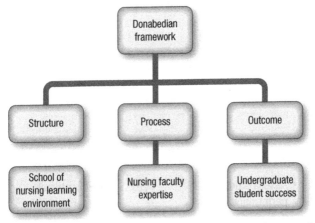

Figure 6.1 Donabedian education process improvement framework.

Micro View: PDSA EPI Framework

The Components of the PDSA Model

- Plan what needs to be accomplished.
- Do whatever it takes to complete the task.
- Study the final product to determine if the intended outcome was met.
- Act in accordance with what you find in the study phase.
- (Moen & Norman, 2010).

All the phases of the PDSA cycle continuously interact to attain and maintain quality (Moen, 2009). This process is easily applied to assessment of competence for a specific skill and provides a structure and foundation for quality (Figure 6.2).

Fast Facts

"It is impossible to fix or improve what is not understood. Direct observations are key to uncovering targets for interventions" (Roehrs, 2018, p. 196).

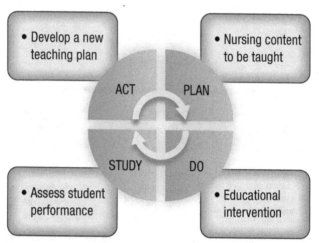

Figure 6.2 PDSA education process improvement model.

Evidence-Based Teaching

Baily et al. (2017) used a PDSA model in a global classroom to teach end-of-life competencies with enhanced educational experiences for all students as the result. The PDSA was used to guide the curriculum!

DEFINITIONS FOR EDUCATION PROCESS IMPROVEMENT

Donabedian EPI Definitions

Structure: Structure indicates the teaching environment, the qualifications of the faculty, and the administrative practices that support educating students (Ayanian & Markel, 2016; Donabedian, 2005). Structure answers questions such as:

- How do "they" see the impact of education on the expected outcomes?
- Do you have the resources necessary for a successful program?
- Are the nurse educators competent in the content being taught?

Process: The ability to successfully and competently complete a technical skill and provide safe patient care. Patient outcomes can sometimes be an indicator of quality; it may benefit you and your faculty to analyze the process used to provide care. By reviewing the process, you can also assess adherence to standards of care. Case studies, simulations, or clinical scenarios are examples of how to create an adequate "sample" to assess quality. This allows for generalizable assumptions about the performance of the learner (Donabedian, 2005).

When it comes to assessing each learning activity, "empirical standards come from actual practice..." (Donabedian, 2005, p. 702). When teaching, the practice standards must be evidence-based and all assessment tools must be aligned with these standards to make the tool valid (Downing, 2003). In addition, most often, the assessment tool is a criterion-based assessment; it measures the individual's performance against a practice standard (Waltz et al., 2016).

Outcome: "How precise do estimates of quality have to be?" (Donabedian, 2005, p. 715). Grading rubrics can measure outcomes. A rubric makes the outcomes' metrics clear to both the educator as well as the student.

Deming PDSA Definitions

"To determine if improvement occurs, the change needs to be studied and measured" (Roehrs, 2018, p. 196). The Deming PDSA cycle guides the process of educating both individuals and groups of students in assessing their knowledge and competence (Table 6.1).

Plan: When establishing the education plan, determine what needs to be taught along with clearly stated outcomes to provide a foundation for what is measured and how to determine success (Roehrs, 2018). This starting point in the PDSA cycle sets the objectives and answers questions such as:

- Who will provide this instruction?
- Who is the target audience for this learning activity?

- Where is the best location for this learning activity (i.e., lecture hall, simulation lab)?
- When will this activity be presented? (Moen, 2009)
- What standards of practice will student performance be measured?
- What is the expected outcome(s) or passing grade?

This plan clarifies what the educator is striving to improve.

Do: This step refers to the actions or plan carried out by the educator or instructor. The analysis of student performance starts at this step (Moen, 2009) and is measured using a criterion-based assessment tool that measures each student's performance against a practice standard (Waltz et al., 2016).

Study: This step takes a very pragmatic approach to measuring and assessing the action of the student's performance. The student's performance is compared to what the instructor defined in the plan step of this process. Critical to the learning process, feedback may be given to the participant (Eraut, 2004) during this study phase.

Act: After evaluation, the educator's actions help to improve those behaviors that did not meet the expected

Table 6.1

Application of Deming's PDSA Cycle in Nursing Education	
Deming Cycle	**Nursing Education Action**
Plan	Plan the education activity with clear expectations of the expected outcomes
Do	Teach the content as planned
Study	Check the competence of the student through a formative assessment
Act	Based on the student's outcome from the assessment, reteach/remediate as required

Source: Moen, R. D. (2009). Foundation and history of the PDSA cycle. *Asian Network for Quality Conference in Tokyo,* September 17, 2009.

outcome (Roehrs, 2018). The evaluation of the student's performance determines the necessary next steps. Next steps could be remediation and a new revised cycle starting at the Plan step again (Moen, 2009). It could also mean passing the student because their performance met the criteria established in the Plan.

HISTORY OF PROCESS IMPROVEMENT

Born in 1919 in Beirut, Lebanon, Avedis Donabedian, MD, established a quality framework that is foundational to understanding how quality and healthcare work in tandem. In 1966, and later refreshed in 2005, Dr. Donabedian shared his model for assessing quality healthcare, which consisted of three parts: structure, process, and outcome. In his 1966 publication, *Evaluating the Quality of Medical Care,* which was "one of the most frequently cited public health articles" (Ayanian & Markel, 2016, p. 205), Dr. Donabedian proposed applying this "triad" to healthcare. Donabedian's work later influenced the Institute of Medicine's 1990 publications called *Medicare: A Strategy for Quality Assurance* and *Crossing the Quality Chasm* (Ayanian & Markel, 2016).

W. Edwards Deming was born in 1900 (Best & Neuhauser, 2005), became an engineer and mathematician (Valeras, 2019), and is most often associated with the PDSA cycle. His work can be traced back to the scientific method of Galileo in 1610, the Shewart Cycle of 1939, and the Japanese PDCA cycle of both 1951 and 1980. Deming refined this cycle from 1986 through 1993 (Moen, 2009). Much of his teaching was directed to the business industry. It was adopted by healthcare quality improvement teams when Deming became a patient himself and realized that while nurses were well-educated and doing the best job possible, it was the system that needed to improve its quality (Best & Neuhauser, 2005).

"Institute leadership. The aim of supervision should be to help people and machines and gadgets to do a better job" (one of Deming's 14 points of management; Best & Neuhauser, 2005, p. 311).

THEORETICAL UNDERPINNINGS OF EDUCATION PROCESS IMPROVEMENT

Both Deming and Donabedian provide a foundation for quality improvement in healthcare. Donabedian's Structure, Process, Outcomes framework offers a macro view for how infrastructures, like a school of nursing, can be organized so a sound process supports quality nursing education. Deming, on the other hand, provides a more detailed approach to actual teaching strategies. These strategies follow the Plan, Do, Study, Act cycle and support the translation of evidence-based information to the teaching practice of nursing educators. Together, this quality improvement approach to nursing education is predictable and outcomes-driven and can effectively educate the nursing workforce of the future.

6.1 Example Vignette

The undergraduate program has a structure in place that requires all technical skills taught to all nursing students to be evidence-based practice standards as defined by nursing and healthcare regulatory bodies such as the Centers for Medicare & Medicaid Services (Donabedian Model: Structure). Expert clinical faculty (Donabedian Model: Process) are planning for the sophomore student experience in the simulation laboratory. They are establishing the teaching strategy

(continued)

(continued)

and grading rubric to measure the student performance for indwelling urinary catheter insertion (Donabedian Model: Outcome).

Each student is provided with all the requirements to prepare for this class in the course syllabus, along with the grading rubric. This includes the necessary reading in the textbook and the required self-paced learning activity hosted on the college learning management system (Deming: Plan). On the day of the actual class in the simulation laboratory, all necessary supplies are made available so each student can practice inserting a urinary catheter into a task trainer. Instructors prepare to evaluate each student's performance using a criterion-based assessment tool developed directly from the evidence (Deming: Do). Each student then completes the procedure for insertion of an indwelling urinary catheter while the instructor measures their performance by direct observation. The assessment tool serves as a road map for accuracy and competence for completing each step correctly (Deming: Study). Based on the individual performance, each student is evaluated for competence for this skill and the next step is determined based on the outcome of completing the procedure correctly (Deming: Act).

THE STUDENT INVOLVED IN PROCESS IMPROVEMENT

Provided that the assessment tool is valid and reliable, students can serve as peer assessors or even evaluate themselves (Eraut, 2004). With specific direction and parameters, students can complete a PDSA cycle without an educator and be successful. The same guidelines apply even if the students are teaching themselves or each other. The content to be taught and assessed is evidence-based, with an assessment tool that is reliable and valid.

SUMMARY

As the Donabedian framework proclaims, structure is the foundation that supports the process and results in outcomes. When aligning this framework to nursing education, consider the Structure: the administrative foundation; Process: how and where the program is delivered, and the expertise and competence of the faculty; and Outcomes: how success is measured and determined (Donabedian, 2005). Simply stated, the components of the PDSA Model include: Plan what needs to be accomplished in the learning environment; Do whatever it takes to complete the task; Study the final product in the form of an assessment to determine if the intended outcome was met; and Act in accordance with what you find in the study phase (Moen & Norman 2010).

REFERENCES

American Association of Colleges of Nursing. (2019). *AACN's vision for academic nursing white paper.* Executive Summary, January.

Ayanian, J. Z., & Markel, H. (2016). Donabedian's lasting framework for health care quality. *New England Journal of Medicine, 375*(3), 205–207. https://doi.org/10.1056/NEJMp1605101

Baily, C., Hewison, A., Orr, S., & Baernholdt, M. (2017). Learning about end-of-life care in nursing—A global classroom educational innovation. *Journal of Nursing Education, 56*(11), 688–691. http://dx.doi.org.proxy1.lib.tju.edu/10.3928/01484834-20171020-10

Best, M., & Neuhauser, D. (2005). W Edwards Deming: Father of quality management, patient and composer. *Quality Safety Health Care, 14,* 310–312. https://doi.org/10.1136/qshc.2005.015289

Donabedian, A. (2005). Evaluating the quality of medical care. *The Milbank Quarterly, 83*(4), 691–729. https://doi.org/10.1111/j.1468-0009.2005.00397.x

Downing, S. M. (2003). Validity: On the meaningful interpretation of assessment data. *Medical Education, 37*(9), 830–830. https://doi.org/10.1046/j.1365-2923.2003.01594.x

Eraut, M. (2004). A wider perspective on assessment. *Medical Education, 38,* 800–804. https://doi.org/10.1111/j.1365-2929.2004.01930.x

Moen, R. D. (2009). Foundation and history of the PDSA cycle. *Asian Network for Quality Conference in Tokyo,* September 17, 2009.

Moen, R. D., & Norman, C. L. (2010). Circling back. *Quality Progress, 43*(11), 22–28.

Roehrs, S. (2018). Building of profound knowledge. *Current Problems in Pediatric and Adolescent Health Care, 48,* 196–197. https://doi.org/10.1016/j.cppeds.2018.08.013

Valeras, A. S. (2019). Quality improvement in a complex world. *American Psychological Association, 37*(4), 352–353. https://doi.org/10.1037/fsh0000454

Waltz, C. F., Strickland, O. L., & Lenz, E. R. (2016). *Measurement in nursing and health research* (5th ed.). Springer Publishing Company.

7

Competency-Based Education for Undergraduate Nursing Curricula

Dawn M. Goodolf

"Great things come from hard work and perseverance."
—Kobe Bryant

OBJECTIVES

- Discuss competency-based education (CBE) and its relevance to undergraduate nursing education.
- Apply the recommendations from the American Association for Colleges of Nursing's (AACN) new vision for academic nursing in developing a competency-based undergraduate nursing curriculum.
- Apply CBE active learning strategies to undergraduate curriculums.

INTRODUCTION

The call for transformation in nursing education has been a priority over the past decade and has been gaining increased attention. There is a call to prepare graduates for the rapidly changing healthcare environment, which requires the delivery of healthcare in increasingly technologically enhanced settings. The American Association for Colleges of Nursing (AACN, 2019a) recently created an Essentials Taskforce that is proposing new guidelines to transform the vision for nursing education.

Currently, entry-level nursing education emphasizes preparing graduates for hospital acute care. The AACN Essentials Taskforce recognized that the healthcare system is growing more complex and there is increasing movement of care to the community. Therefore, entry-level professional nurses need competencies in team-based and coordinated care across a variety of clinical agencies.

The AACN Essentials Taskforce recommends entry-level professional nursing education prepare a generalist for practice across the lifespan and continuum of care. Nursing competencies need to provide guidance in how/what faculty teach, direction on what faculty expect of students, and frameworks for performance assessment across all spheres of care and professional practice (AACN, 2019a).

The current model of clinical nursing education cannot control learning experiences for each student. There may be planned hours of time, but there is no assurance that all students have equitable experiences or that competencies are achieved. Moving to a competency-based model would foster intentionality by defining competencies and associated attributes, methods for achievement, and outcome measurement (AACN, 2019a).

The AACN Essentials Taskforce is proposing a new vision for nursing education that will create competencies and outcomes expected for all entry-level BSN graduates. The AACN Essentials Taskforce recommends entry-level professional nursing education prepare a generalist for practice across the lifespan and continuum of care. Table 7.1 describes the four areas of practice for the entry-level generalist nurse.

Expected competencies for generalist entry-level nursing practice will include observable and measurable competencies across the four spheres of care. The undergraduate curriculum will need to include clinical experiences within appropriate sites that reflect the four spheres of care and include combinations of experiences in acute care, ambulatory, primary care, long-term care, palliative care, and any other relevant settings. The undergraduate curriculum should also include immersion experiences encompassing one or more of the four spheres of care near the end of the degree program for all entry-level students. These experiences are designed to integrate learning into clinical practice, increase care competencies, provide continuity, and increase confidence in performing as a generalist nurse (AACN, 2019a). Therefore, the completion of the undergraduate degree will be driven by the

Table 7.1

AACN Essentials Taskforce's Four Areas of Practice for Generalists

Disease prevention/ promotion of health and well-being	The promotion of physical and mental health in all patients as well as management of minor acute and intermittent care needs of generally healthy patients
Chronic disease care	Management of chronic diseases and prevention of negative sequela
Regenerative or restorative care	Critical/trauma care, complex acute care, acute exacerbations of chronic conditions, and treatment of physiologically unstable patients that generally requires care in a mega-acute care institution
Hospice/palliative/ supportive care	

Source: American Association of Colleges of Nursing. (2019a). *AACN's vision for academic nursing.* https://www.aacnnursing.org/Portals/42/News/White -Papers/Vision-Academic-Nursing.pdf

achievement of the identified competencies as well as the designated number of credit hours.

To level the expected competency outcomes for the undergraduate curriculum, the AACN Essentials Task Force (2019b) has recommended the following 10 domains and descriptors (Table 7.2).

Table 7.2

AACN's Ten Domains and Descriptors

Domain	Descriptor
Knowledge for Nursing Practice	Integration, translation, and application of established and evolving disciplinary nursing knowledge and ways of knowing, as well as knowledge from other disciplines. This distinguishes the practice of professional nursing and forms the basis for clinical judgment and innovation in nursing practice.
Person-Centered Care	Provision of holistic and just care, which is respectful, compassionate, and coordinated. This reflects the differences, preferences, values, needs, and resources of the person or designee as the source of control and full partner. Person-centered care is informed by evidence and supports the achievement of positive health outcomes.
Population Health	Engagement in partnerships to support and improve equitable population health outcomes.
Scholarship for Nursing Practice	The generation, synthesis, translation, application, and dissemination of knowledge to improve health and transform healthcare.
Quality and Safety	Employment of established and emerging principles of safety science and quality in nursing and healthcare as an essential component of practice.
Interprofessional Partnerships	Intentionally working together across professions and with care team members, patients, families, and communities to optimize care, enhance the experience, improve outcomes, and reduce costs.

(continued)

Table 7.2

AACN's Ten Domains and Descriptors *(Continued)*	
Domain	**Descriptor**
System-Based Practice	Responding to and leading within complex systems of healthcare.
Informatics and Healthcare Technologies	The use of informatics, which encompasses healthcare technologies and information communication technologies, to manage and improve the delivery of nursing and healthcare services in accordance with best practice and professional and regulatory standards.
Professionalism	Formation and cultivation of a sustainable professional nursing identity, accountability, perspective, collaborative disposition, and comportment that reflects nursing's characteristics, norms, and values
Personal, Professional, and Leadership Development	Participation in activities and self-reflection that foster personal health, resilience, and well-being, lifelong learning, and support the acquisition of nursing expertise and assertion of leadership.

These potential domains and descriptors provide the structure and framework for the competency outcomes for those graduating from an entry into practice curriculum and provide a strong foundational basis for new graduates as they transition into practice.

QUALITY AND SAFETY FOR NURSES

Quality and Safety Education for Nurses (QSEN) also addresses nursing competencies needed to ensure quality and safety of patient care. Using the Institute of Medicine's (2003) competencies for nursing, QSEN faculty have defined pre-licensure and graduate quality and safety competencies for nursing, and proposed goals for the knowledge, skills, and attitudes to be developed in nursing pre-licensure programs for each. Many of these competencies are already being addressed in the healthcare setting, but they need to utilize similar language in our competency statements and be further integrated into everyday practice (Hunt, 2012).

Six QSEN Competencies

- Patient-Centered Care
- Teamwork & Collaboration
- Evidence-Based Practice
- Quality Improvement
- Safety
- Informatics

Each competency contains expectations relating to knowledge, skills, and attitudes to be achieved. The QSEN competencies are ranked beginner, intermediate, and advanced learning objectives for integration across the learning curriculum (Forneris et al., 2012). By the time students graduate, they should achieve all competencies and be able to utilize them in their professional practice (Hunt, 2012).

CBE IN THE UNDERGRADUATE CLASSROOM

Nurses need to base their thinking on situations, evidence, and standards that support their daily decisions. The focus on teaching competency-based education (CBE) is to assist the student to think like a nurse, which means the critical thinking needs to be deliberate, skillful, responsible, and thoughtful (Caputi, 2018).

Once the decision has been made to incorporate a competency-based curriculum, faculty must determine or identify the organizational framework for the curriculum.

Steps in Developing/Identifying an Organizational Framework

- Develop the concept categories
- Select and develop the concepts
- Select exemplars

- Course development
  (Giddens et al., 2020).

This will require educators to teach conceptually using active teaching strategies to enhance student understanding and clinical application.

The overarching goal of conceptual teaching is to help the student build a conceptual understanding of nursing that is transferable to a variety of health conditions and competencies (Giddens et al., 2020). While in the classroom, faculty must first teach the concept or content, beginning with a formal concept overview for each concept in the curriculum. Each concept should contain designated exemplars that link the concept to a patient or situational context to promote application. The faculty should continually make connections and build on previous understanding of the concept. Finally, it is encouraged to utilize a variety of student-centered teaching strategies to foster collaborative learning.

In a concept-based curriculum, the major nursing concepts are taught with a focus on application within nursing practice. Content must be presented based on patient situations that launch a cascade of details about the concepts, related concepts, health conditions and related problems, and the total patient picture (Giddens et al., 2020). Understanding the total patient picture increases competency.

CONCEPT PRESENTATION

Concept presentation means each concept should be taught formally (Giddens et al., 2020). The sequencing of concept presentations depends on the nursing curriculum. Faculty should utilize a template for concept presentation across all courses. Once this template has been developed, faculty should consider which learning activities to use for the presentation. Developing a lesson plan for concept presentation creates a fair and purposeful learning experience for students (Giddens et al., 2020). All lesson plans should balance faculty-led and student-centered activities. Other interrelated concepts emerge when the concept is applied to a specific clinical context.

EXEMPLARS

An exemplar is an example of a health condition or situation in which the concept would be present. After the concept presentation, exemplars assist the student's understanding of the concept. Exemplars provide contextual application of knowledge gained in the classroom and may be reinforced in the clinical setting (Giddens et al., 2020). Faculty should select exemplars based on evidence and data to expose students to the most important and prevalent content (Johnston, 2017). Teaching exemplars give students an opportunity to understand the concept more deeply.

Teaching an excess of exemplars results in content saturation, making students lose sight of the concept (Giddens et al., 2020). It is the hope of faculty that students will be able to apply the concepts to a variety of new exemplars, even those that have not been covered in the class (Dailey, 2016).

SITUATIONAL LEARNING

Situational learning helps students to understand how lessons apply to practice (Giddens et al., 2020). One of the most common methods of accomplishing this in the classroom is through the use of case studies. Case studies focus on a single situation relevant to the topic being studied, and unfolding case studies present a situation over time (Giddens et al., 2020).

Standardized virtual patients are fictional characters that also support learning throughout the curriculum. Students become familiar with the virtual patient, and their health history, family situation, and living conditions, which faculty may utilize throughout the curriculum (Giddens et al., 2020).

STUDENT-CENTERED LEARNING STRATEGIES

A variety of teaching strategies promote student-centered conceptual learning. These strategies actively engage students, focus on a clinical situation, and require students to think critically (Giddens et al., 2020). Faculty should promote guided questions that require the student to draw on previous experiences to foster their ability in applying what they learned to new situations.

Active learning strategies that may be incorporated into the CBE classroom:

- Flipping the classroom
- Case studies
- Unfolding case studies
- Virtual patient scenarios
- Gaming and game-based response systems
- Debate
- Guided questions
- Vignettes
- NCLEX-style questioning
- Clinical judgment exercises
- Peer teaching
- Collaborative assessment

Fast Facts

An effective active learning strategy that may be incorporated into the CBE classroom is flipping the classroom. The learning is accountable to explore information in a self-directed manner outside of class (Brewer & Movahedazarhouligh, 2018).

CBE IN THE UNDERGRADUATE CLINICAL SETTING

Clinical settings provide an opportunity to extend and deepen the student's conceptual understanding as they directly experience concepts associated with the nursing profession as they appear in practice (Giddens et al., 2020). Benner et al. (2010) recognized the importance of educating nurses to be lifelong expert learners and reflective practitioners; nursing students are entering a practice that will only become more complex with time. Historically, students were primarily educated in an acute care setting; however, it is recommended students be prepared for a diverse role in non-traditional settings (AACN, 2019a; Giddens et al., 2020).

Conceptual learning may be achieved through a combination of direct patient care experiences (DPC) and focused learning activities (FLAs). DPC experiences are learning activities that can be completed in a hospital or community setting while providing patient care. FLAs are also completed in an acute care or community setting but intentionally focus on concepts that foster the development of clinical judgment (Fletcher & Meyer, 2016). Integrating these lessons and experiences throughout the curriculum provides a strong educational foundation as students enter their final practicum experience in their final semester of the program (Fletcher & Meyer, 2016).

Clinical assignments can be structured so the student is responsible for planning, implementing, and evaluating care for one or more patients. This would require the student to demonstrate competence in patient care management. In a concept-based curriculum, the application of concepts is incorporated through written assignments, discussions with faculty members, and post conference(Giddens et al., 2020).

Faculty should create a lesson plan for the clinical setting similar to that of the classroom setting. Specific clinical assignments should be incorporated into the course syllabus so students clearly understand clinical expectations (Giddens et al., 2020). Written assignments can be incorporated into clinical rotations. The purpose of assignments is to promote the understanding of concepts, promote thinking and clinical judgment, promote reflection, and provide meaningful feedback and evaluation (Giddens et al., 2020).

Fast Facts

Bilik et al. (2020) completed a university study that demonstrated that web-based concept mapping increased critical thinking skills in students.

Active learning strategies that may be incorporated into the CBE clinical setting:

- Concept maps
- Concept analyses
- Case studies
- Case presentations
- Collaborative clinical assignments
- Nursing care plans
- Teaching plans
- Reflective journals
- Guided worksheets.

The role of clinical faculty is to help students gain higher-order thinking skills during the clinical experience. Faculty should use open-ended questions to explain their thinking, rationale, and connection to concepts (Giddens et al., 2020).

SIMULATION LEARNING

Simulation in undergraduate nursing curricula provides realistic student-centered learning opportunities by incorporating virtual reality and allowing for immediate feedback. Using simulation, the student can become competent, reflect on their skills, and improve performance, which will ultimately be transferable into the healthcare setting (Kiernan, 2018). Simulated experiences provide the opportunity for faculty to observe for needed changes in student behavior.

Debriefing after the simulated experience permits facilitated reflection and is essential for performance improvement

(Eppich & Cheng, 2015). Debriefing allows the student to reflect on their own actions and provide rationales for their decisions. Team-based debriefing offers opportunities for students to reflect and collaborate in a transformative learning process (Fletcher & Meyer, 2016). Effective debriefing is a crucial part of the simulated experience, but despite the increased use of simulation in the undergraduate curriculum, many educators have little or no previous formal training in debriefing and struggle to facilitate the process effectively. A debriefing script in all simulated experiences can foster the student-centered learning experience (Eppich & Cheng, 2015).

Educators need to develop simulation experiences using evidence-based approaches to foster deliberate practice. This focused approach will develop clinical competence and confidence for nursing students (Kiernan, 2018). A student's confidence can be built through the use of simulation, which leads to increased knowledge and fosters critical thinking.

7.1 Example Vignette

Nursing faculty have an important role in ensuring students develop skills that can be used in a variety of clinical settings. Clinical adjunct faculty may be unsure of how to evaluate students using a competency-based evaluation system. Iglesias-Parra et al. (2015) developed and validated an instrument based on the Nursing Interventions Classification (NIC) to evaluate clinical competence of students pursuing a nursing degree. Through their research, they found that evaluating clinical skills utilizing the NIC provides a framework for reliable and valid assessment that allows for the description of interventions in a standardized and comparable way (Iglesias-Parra et al., 2015). Utilizing a standardized tool for all faculty will assist in guiding the learning process for both students and faculty in a variety of clinical settings.

BOX 7.1 EVIDENCE-BASED TEACHING PRACTICE

Yockey and Henry (2019) explored sources of anxiety for nursing students, as it was related to simulation experiences and progression through the nursing curriculum. Excessive anxiety has been known to impair learning and performance. Based on the top anxiety sources from the study, recommendations to lessen simulation anxiety included: Student role:

- Base expectations on simulation objectives and not outside of student abilities.
- Verify that students understand the faculty and student roles.
- Limit the number of observers.
- Allow private review of simulation video for personal reflection.
- Consider discussion of anticipated plan of care as part of the prebriefing.
- Create an expectation of positive peer support and engagement.
- Remediate in private.

Fear of Making a Mistake:

- Provide faculty training for facilitation of skills and delivery of timely, meaningful feedback.
- Focus feedback on preventing future errors.
- Allow practice of expected skills, including a "practice simulation."
- Create a safe learning environment.
- Include a clinical reasoning aspect in simulation preparation to allow reflection on possible unknown client situations.
- Have observers in separate area of scenario performance.
- Support performance expectations and establish a trusting relationship.

SUMMARY

Undergraduate nursing curriculum can use traditional and non-traditional teaching-learning methods to incorporate CBE by establishing a framework based on goals and objectives. Essential competencies needed to achieve the goals and prepare entry-level nurses can be derived from standards that include multiple clinical learning environments and innovative teaching strategies. Cognitively understanding concepts and applying them to clinical practice safely with professionalism can be achieved through thoughtful planning and evaluation.

REFERENCES

American Association of Colleges of Nursing. (2019a). *AACN's vision for academic nursing*. https://www.aacnnursing.org/Portals/42/News/White-Papers/Vision-Academic-Nursing.pdf

American Association of Colleges of Nursing. (2019b). *Draft of domains and descriptors*. https://www.aacnnursing.org/Portals/42/Downloads/Essentials/Essentials-Revision-Domains-Descriptors.pdf

Benner, P., Sutphen, M., & Day, L. V. (2010). *Educating nurses: A call for radical transformation*. Josey-Bass.

Bilik, O., Kankaya, E. A., & Deveci, Z. (2020). Effects of web-based concept mapping education on students' concept mapping and critical thinking skills: A double blind, randomized, controlled study. *Nurse Education Today, 86*, 1–6. https://doi.org/10.1016/j.nedt.2019.104312

Brewer, R., & Movahedazarhouligh, S. (2018). Successful stories and conflicts: A literature review on the effectiveness of flipped learning in higher education. *Wiley Journal of Computer Assisted earning, 34*(4), 409–416. https://doi.org/10.1111/jcal.12250

Caputi, L. (2018). *Think like a nurse: A handbook*. Windy City Publishers.

Dailey, J. (2016). *The concept-based curriculum: Key points for a transition*. Elsevier Academic Consulting Group. White Paper. Erickson, H.L.

Eppich, W., & Cheng, A. (2015). Promoting excellence and reflective learning in simulation (PEARLS): Development and rationale for a blended approach to health care simulation debriefing. *Simulation in Healthcare, 10*(2), 106–115. https://doi.org/10.1097/SIH.0000000000000072

Fletcher, K., & Meyer, M. (2016). Coaching model + clinical playbook = transformative learning. *Journal of Professional Nursing, 32*(2), 121–129. https://doi.org/10.1016/j.profnurs.2015.09.001

Fornereris, S., Crownover, J., Dorsey, L., Leahy, N., Maas, N., Wong, L., Zabriskie, A., & Zavertnik, J. (2012). Integrating QSEN and ACES: An NLN simulation leader project. *Nursing Education Perspectives, 33*(3), 184–186. https://doi.org/10.5480/1536-5026-33.3.184

Giddens, J., Caputi, L., & Rodgers, B. (2020). *Mastering concept-based teaching. A guide for nurse educators* (2nd ed.). Elsevier.

Hunt, D. (2012). QSEN competencies: A bridge to practice. *Nursing Made Incredibly Easy, 10*(5), 1–3. https://doi.org/10.1097/01.NME.0000418040.92006.70

Iglesias-Parra, M. R. (2015). Design of a competency-based evaluation model for clinical nursing practicum, based on standardized language systems: Psychometric validation study. *Journal of Nursing Scholarship, 47*(4), 371–376. https://doi.org/10.1111/jnu.12140

Institute of Medicine. (2003). *Health professions education: A bridge to quality*. National Academic Press.

Johnston, D. (2017). *Navigating the move to concept-based curriculum. Part 1: Designing a concept-based curriculum*. https://www.atitesting.com/docs/default-source/research/navigating_the_move_to_cbc.pdf?sfvrsn=97e106e9_0

Kiernan, L. (2018). Evaluating competence and confidence using simulation technology. *Nursing, 48*(10), 45–52. https://doi.org/10.1097/01.NURSE.0000545022.36908.f3

Yockey, J., & Henry, M. (2019). Simulation anxiety across the curriculum. *Clinical Simulation in Nursing, 29*(C), 29–37. https://doi.org/10.1016/j.ecns.2018.12.004

8

Competency-Based Education for Graduate (MSN) Nursing Curricula

Catherine Johnson and Denise Lucas

"If we know why we are learning and if the reason fits our needs as we perceive them, we will learn quickly and deeply."

— Malcolm Knowles

OBJECTIVES

- Demonstrate understanding of adult learning principles impacting graduate nursing programs.
- Apply elements of competency-based education (CBE) key framework elements with adult learners in online graduate Master's of Science in Nursing (MSN) programs.
- Apply CBE teaching-learning strategies to online education.

INTRODUCTION

In the past 20 years, nursing and all other healthcare professions have been challenged to use evidence as a basis for practice and to better educate its members in the use of scientific theory and research. In response, graduate nursing education has expanded opportunities for nurses to continue their education and demonstrate a level of readiness in meeting professional competencies (Anema & McCoy, 2010).

Hybrid or fully online education made this expansion possible and are the common formats for graduate nursing programs. Graduate Master's of Science in Nursing (MSN) programs that focus on nursing specialties such as nursing executive, clinical nurse leader, nursing informatics, nursing education, and forensic nursing, to name a few, are thriving more than ever in online platforms. Many nurses will choose to remain in their communities and become leaders in providing needed healthcare services. In doing so, the nursing profession will be able to meet the demand for increased healthcare services to underserved populations identified in the Institute of Medicine (IOM) Future of Nursing (2010) report.

ONLINE LEARNING PEDAGOGY

Malcolm Knowles (1970), a leader in the development of adult learning theories, asserted program faculty should actively engage adult learners in learning activities that must be learner-centered, self-directed, experiential, and directly applicable to the student's own perception of importance. These principles were based upon Knowles's (1984) understanding of adult development and how this impacts their learning. These adult development concepts are summarized in Table 8.1

The adult learning principles reflect many of the competency-based education (CBE) concepts that come into play as faculty develop online graduate MSN nursing programs.

Table 8.1

Malcolm Knowles Adult Learning Principles	
Self-Concept	As adults mature, their self-concept moves from being dependent to being self-directed.
Resources for Learning	As adults mature, they accumulate life experiences which increasingly become their primary resource for learning.
Readiness to Learn	As adults mature, their readiness to learn becomes oriented to tasks of their social roles.
Application of Learning	As adults mature, their time perspective changes from postponing application of new knowledge to immediacy of application.
Problem-Focused	As adults mature, their orientation to learning shifts from subject centered to problem centered.
Motivation to Learn	As adults mature, their orientation to learning shifts from external to internal motivation.

Source: Knowles, M. S. (1984). *Andragogy in action.* Jossey-Bass.

In addition to learning these concepts, faculty must examine their perspective about the faculty-student relationship. Many graduate nursing faculty have worked in undergraduate courses and interacted with younger students, which requires a supervisory role with highly structured courses, assignments, and interactions. Undergraduate faculty have traditionally been seen as the "Sage on the Stage" and have presented lectures from podiums in large lecture halls, providing information to students with little opportunity for discussion or questions.

When working with adult students through Learning Management Systems (LMS), online graduate MSN nursing faculty must differently conceptualize their role and their approach to learning. Applying adult learning principles to the creation of a supportive climate includes a learner-centered approach to scholarly activities and assignments that enhance learning and support achievement of competency-based outcomes.

CREATING A SUPPORTIVE LEARNING ENVIRONMENT

Positive learning environments for adults address both their physical and psychological needs (Knowles, 1984). In online programs, the physical environment is structured through the features of the LMS. But graduate nursing faculty can tailor this environment through creative announcements, discussion boards, and other activities that make the adult learner excited to join this active environment. Welcome videos produced by the faculty set a friendly tone for students in the first days of the course and walk students through the course features and elements. Introduction discussion boards ask students to create their own videos or creative means of introducing themselves to the class.

All of these are examples of efforts made by course faculty to meet the physical as well as psychological needs of the adult student to feel safe, secure, and acknowledged. Knowles (1970) emphasized that adults "learn better when they feel supported rather than judged or threatened." Faculty members can be the creator of supportive climates within the online environment that assist adult learners in achieving the competencies and outcomes desired.

SUPPORTING ADULT LEARNER INVOLVEMENT

Faculty must recognize that they are working with experienced and competent adults (Knowles, 1984). This basic understanding is critical for effective communication with adult learners. Online communication relies on the written word to convey complex information and concerns between faculty and students, as well as among students. Online communication can create barriers to building trust and feelings of safety despite all parties' best efforts. Faculty teaching online should be extremely aware of the positive and negative impact of their communication and feedback to students at all times and be prepared to respond positively should students misunderstand. Adult learners are often labeled as resistant or contentious when instead, they may not feel supported or safe. Faculty must be aware of the needs of adult learners and provide understanding and support.

Knowles (1984) encourages faculty to be inclusive and involve students in the development of assignments and other learning opportunities. Adults learn through connection of new knowledge with their values and experiences. Through a "general to specific" approach, start with an overview of a topic or learning objective and then move into the more specific details of the information or skills application (Knowles, 1984). By connecting with what the adult learner already knows, they will feel more recognized and competent at a certain level of application. From this platform, they can build new knowledge and skill competency. Faculty who seek to build this confidence and acknowledgment of prior knowledge and skill will facilitate the adult learner's higher achievement.

Crosswalk: CBE Key Framework Elements With Knowles' Characteristics of Adult Learners

This crosswalk compares Gruppen et al.'s (2016) four Concept-Based Framework elements with five key adult learner characteristics identified by Knowles (1984).

	Outcome Focus	Abilities Emphasis	Learner-Centered	No Focus on Time
Active Participation		X	X	X
Individual Differences		X	X	X
Experience has a Role	X	X	X	
Immediate & Relevant Impact	X	X	X	
Problem Centered	X	X	X	

LEARNING MANAGEMENT SYSTEMS (LMS)

U.S. colleges and universities are now establishing a worldwide presence through nursing graduate degrees using learning management systems (LMS) such as Blackboard, Moodle, Canvas, and other platforms. Graduate MSN nursing programs compete with nursing programs not only in their geographic region, but also with all other online graduate nursing programs around the United States. This competition challenges colleges and schools of nursing to provide effective, high-quality online programs focused on national competencies and role definitions. Colleges and schools of nursing must create graduate nursing programs that appeal to nurses of all ages. This includes providing sophisticated LMS that are easy to operate and fully integrated with online resources. LMS are designed to support planning, implementation, and evaluation of a learning process. These new systems often provide graduate students the same services students formally find on campus, including online libraries, writing centers, graduate nursing advising, and career counseling. LMS are the framework on which the workflow of a graduate nursing course can be built.

Using LMS, nursing faculty can share their expectations for the course through posted course profiles and course schedules; make assignments and grade them; share content, including faculty-developed materials and open resources such as YouTube videos; and purchase learning materials and programs. Faculty can create group work where students can discuss issues with peers and faculty (discussion boards) as well as co-create documents, presentations, and other learning activities (Wikis). Faculty can communicate through posted videos, VoiceThreads, or conferencing programs such as Zoom or GoToMeeting. All of these efforts should be designed using the lens of adult learning theory. LMS provide the opportunity for faculty to create supportive learning environments and climates for adult learners and enable them to be successful.

Fast Facts

Online learning supports adult learning theory. It promotes student-centered teaching strategies and therefore increased critical thinking and self-assessment (Berkstresser, 2016).

Common Features of LMS

- Developing and sharing content and learning experiences
- Student/student and student/faculty collaboration
- Creating, administering, and scoring exams
- Generating reports regarding student participation for students, faculty, and administrators
- Integration of Internet apps and tools (YouTube, Google Scholar)
- Mobile access using smartphones
- Setting and tracking individual student goals
- Live video conferencing (Zoom, GoToMeeting)
- Integrating with institutions' student information systems

This shift of the educational platform from a face-to-face format to a hybrid or fully online format challenges nursing faculty to build their knowledge of learning theories, strategies, and learning experiences. This shift in educational delivery must build on the 2003 IOM's recommendation for health professional education core competencies, which delineate the following:

1. Provide patient-centered care.
2. Work in interdisciplinary teams.
3. Employ evidence-based practice.
4. Apply quality improvement.
5. Utilize informatics.

Exhibit 8.1

Teaching/Learning Strategies Supporting CBE

CBE Framework Elements	Teaching/Learning Strategies
Active Participation	<ul><li>Case study/vignettes</li><li>Class polling/audience response</li><li>Online conferencing</li><li>Grand rounds</li><li>Group projects</li><li>Concept mapping</li><li>Problem-based learning</li><li>Simulation</li></ul>
Individual Differences	<ul><li>May have more than one learning style (multimodal)<ul><li>Visual</li><li>Auditory</li><li>Read/Write</li><li>Kinesthetic</li><li>Digital</li><li>Analytical</li><li>Reflective</li><li>Intuitive</li></ul></li></ul>
Experience has a role	<ul><li>Learning activities planned</li><li>Increase in skill and complexity</li><li>Students typically possess some clinical expertise in a particular area</li></ul>
Immediate & Relevant Impact	<ul><li>Apply learning to patient care situations</li><li>Enhance communication skills</li><li>Evaluate and utilize evidence-based practice in clinical practice and decision making</li></ul>
Problem-Centered	<ul><li>Case study/dissection</li><li>Grand rounds</li><li>Simulation</li></ul>

Fast Facts

John et al. (2020) studied interprofessional competencies and found most disciplines include competencies in communication, collaboration, and professionalism.

Sinacori (2020) interviewed nursing faculty transitioning from traditional classroom teaching environment to an online program. These nursing faculty identified a need for professional development related to online teaching pedagogy and LMS, and requested a mentorship in transitioning to this new mode of teaching and learning.

The design, implementation, and evaluation of any program or course ensures that CBE is actually being delivered and that the student has an adequate skill set and necessary knowledge level. Due to the variety of MSN programs, teaching/learning strategies may be diverse, encompassed in LMS, and allow room for creativity and customization. Exhibit 8.1 provides teaching/learning strategies that support key elements of CBE.

TEACHING AND EVALUATING OUTCOMES IN AN ONLINE PROGRAM

Technology provided the means for graduate nursing programs to expand through online formats utilizing a variety of LMS activities. There has also been a shift away from traditional didactic approaches toward a system of instruction that incorporates principles of adult learning and CBE.

CBE focuses on building competencies that clearly describe what a student must master to complete a program of study. Program competencies or outcomes define the required mastery for the credentials being earned and are consistent with requirements for certification in the specialty area if available. The program's curriculum provides both content and learning activities designed to support learners in the achievement of these competencies. Course-specific competencies describe mastery of the course content area and are measurable and assessed using valid and reliable methods (Wittmann-Price et al., 2017).

Even though LMS provide easy access to a variety of tools and incorporate them into the CBE curriculum, the faculty's creativity and commitment connect the competency evaluation and the learning activities. Evaluation methods must shift and adapt to online learning environments, which often have students under the auspice of preceptors who provide feedback to both students and faculty. Evaluation tools must be chosen carefully, clearly understood, and usable for a variety of preceptors.

8.1 Example Vignette

A nursing faculty member teaching forensic students in the clinical portion of their program designed preceptor evaluation tools that:

- *are measurable*
- *focus on specific abilities and outcomes for the particular level of the student*
- *identify appropriate and incorporated in patient care*
- *require the identification and incorporation of the latest evidence-based strategies*
- *utilize technology for student log/experience documentation*
- *are useful and easy to understand by a variety of interdisciplinary preceptors in the forensic field*
- *provide the opportunity for evaluation at different levels and time points*

Schools of nursing in undergraduate and graduate programs commonly use simulation in teaching clinical practice skills. Now, technology provides the means to conduct simulations in the online environment. Online simulation integrates theory within the context of practice through well-constructed competency outcomes. Technology connects students and faculty in demonstration of many clinical skills and decision-making processes. Peer-to-peer or instructor-to-student role-playing within a specific practice context can provide students and faculty the opportunity to engage in skill development and evaluation.

LMS provide the tools, such as Zoom meetings, to connect faculty and students. These interactions can be conducted and observed synchronously as well as recorded for formative evaluations, self-assessment, and summative evaluations. These interactions provide experiential learning opportunities that allow for student thinking, planning, and decision-making that supports Knowles's (1984) theory of adult learning. Students can then act, reflect, and self-evaluate, as well as make mistakes, in real time with supervision and feedback from faculty.

Virtual patients are a specific simulation opportunity in which virtual patients are "standardized or simulated patients" who can simulate authentic clinical encounters. These standard patients can be peers, "actors," or the faculty member themselves. Ellaway et al. (2015) described learning activities that can be accomplished using virtual patients, including increasing independent study activities and providing collaborative and synchronous groups. These formats for online simulation activities can further enhance online practice-focused education and help students learn and demonstrate clinical skills online.

BOX 8.1 EVIDENCE-BASED TEACHING PRACTICE

Johnstone and Soares (2014) demonstrate that CBE can fit into existing academic calendars and systems if the four principles below are followed:

There are robust and valid competencies.

Students who learn at different paces are supported in their learning.

Appropriate learning resources are accessible at any time.

Assessments are secure, valid, and reliable.

Technology has provided enhanced environments that allow online students to work independently within an avatar-centered environment and repeat the simulation multiple times as they develop their clinical decision-making skills (Shadow Health; I Human). Students can make mistakes and try new approaches safely. Multiple students can also interact with the "standardized patient" and share experiences to develop a deeper understanding of the clinical decision-making process. Recordings can be made from these interactions to aid the student's learning and, in more formal settings, aid the faculty in competency evaluations.

Technology-enhanced simulations will not replace faculty expertise or real-life experience, but it can enhance online learning and mirror key components to live classrooms. Expanded student interactions with each other and faculty within these virtual worlds is a positive addition to online education (Washburn & Zhou, 2018). Using avatar-based technology, faculty can develop scenarios to suit the needs of their students and expand their skill development.

Key Components of Technology Enhanced Simulations

- Sharing space among students and faculty
- Immediacy of interaction and feedback
- Socialization among students and faculty
- Collaboration among students in problem-solving
- Sharing information in real time
- Easy-to-negotiate user interface
- Clinical problem-solving evaluations by students and faculty

ENHANCING STUDENTS' FLEXIBILITY IN AN ONLINE PROGRAM

- Student-planned orientation
- Online courses
- Hybrid courses

- Eight-week classes
- Flexibility in leave of absence policies
- Online advisors
- Online additional student services (career placement, writing center, library, other virtual tools)
- System to measure and communicate progress throughout course (starfish)
- Financial aid support

8.2 Example Vignette

Individual Responsibility Related to Competency

Nurses have a professional obligation to embrace the idea of life-long learning and become an active participant in this process. Active lifelong learners may do this in a variety of ways that include attending professional conferences and workshops, belonging to and participating in professional nursing organizations, subscribing to professional nursing journals, volunteering for practice improvement opportunities in the workplace, mentoring colleagues, networking regularly, participating in community projects, and of course, continuing their education at an advanced level.

SUMMARY

Developing new master's degrees in nursing based upon emerging needs of the healthcare system most likely will occur in the online environment. All levels of education, from kindergarten to graduate programs, are shifting to ensure there are opportunities for students to demonstrate a significant level of readiness to function once their education is completed (Anema & McCoy, 2010). Utilization of the CBE approach to curriculum design, implementation, and evaluation will facilitate this shift. Adult learners benefit from the

CBE approach and often an online learning environment, as this is consistent with their learning style and personal and professional needs (Hodges et al., 2019). Technology continues to develop and will further expand the capability of nursing programs to teach and evaluate nursing competencies in an online environment. Online graduate MSN students will be able to further their nursing career opportunities and support the provision of needed services to underserved populations, thus meeting the goals for improved health outcomes for all. CBE provides a framework that can guide nursing faculty in their development of online education courses, including learning activities and evaluation methods that are competency based and supportive of adult learning.

Nursing education programs are vast, and there is significant competitiveness among schools for capable students. Institutions and schools of nursing focus on outcomes such as pass rates (when applicable) and graduation rates, student productivity in the forms of publications or projects, and community partner relationships as indicators of success. In order to design effective CBE, nursing faculty must consider four key CBE framework elements that focus on outcomes, emphasis on abilities, student-driven learning activities, and learner-centered environments.

The idea of identifying particular program outcomes is not new; however, making an accurate evaluation of meeting program outcomes may be difficult. In addition, communicating program outcomes to students, using the phrase competency, and defining why competency is important post-graduation is critical. McDonald (2018) cites the importance of communicating this to students early on, in the beginning. Students should complete their program understanding what competency is, what specific objectives their program has assisted them in meeting, and how they transfer this competence to their work setting (Hodges et al., 2019). It is expensive for employers to orient competent or experienced employees, and adding the burden of moving nurses to a level of basic competence so they may be exposed to organizational norms and methods adds to employer costs (Anema & McCoy, 2010).

REFERENCES

Anema, M., & McCoy, J. (2010). *Competency-based nursing education: Guide to achieving outstanding learner outcomes.* Springer Publishing Company.

Berkstresser, K. (2016). The use of online discussions for post-clinical conference. *Nurse Education in Practice, 16*(1), 27–32. https://doi.org/10.1016/j.nepr.2015.06.007

Ellaway, R., Topps, D., Lee, S., & Armson, H. (2015). Virtual patient activity patterns for clinical learning. *Clinical Teacher, 12,* 267–271. http://dx.doi.org/10.1111/tct.12302

Gruppen, L. D., Burkhardt, J. C., Fitzgerald, J. T., Funnell, M., Haftel, H. M., Lypson, M. L., Mullan, P. B., Santen, S. A., Sheets, K. J., Stalburg, K. M., & Vasquez, J. A. (2016). Competency-based education: Programme design and challenges to implementation. *Medical Education, 50,* 532–539. http://dx.doi.org/10.1111/medu.12977

Hodges, A., Jakubisin Konicki, A., Talley, M., Bordelon, C., Holland, A., & Galin, F. (2019). Competency-based education in transitioning nurse practitioner students from education into practice. *Journal of the American Association of Nurse Practitioners, 31*(11), 675–682. http://dx.doi.org/10.1097/JXX.0000000000000327

Institute of Medicine. (2003). *Health professions education: A bridge to quality.* The National Academies Press. https://doi.org/10.17226/10681

Institute of Medicine. (2010). *The future of nursing: Leading change, advancing health.* The National Academies Press.

John, M. S., Tong, B., Li, E., & Wilbur, K. (2020). Competency-based education frameworks across Canadian health professions and implications for multisource feedback. *Journal of Allied Health, 49*(1), e1–e11.

Johnstone, S. M., & Soares, L. (2014). Principles for developing competency-based education programs. *Change: The Magazine of Higher Learning, 46*(2), 12–19.

Knowles, M. S. (1970). *The modern practice of adult learning.* Prentice Hall.

Knowles, M. S. (1984). *Andragogy in action*. Jossey-Bass.

McDonald, M. (2018). *The nurse educator's guide to assessing learning outcomes* (4th ed.). Jones & Bartlett Learning.

Sinacori, B. (2020). How nurse educators perceive the transition from the traditional classroom to the online environment: A qualitative inquiry. *Nursing Education Perspectives, 41*(1), 16–19. http://dx.doi.org/10.1097/01.NEP.0000000000000490

Washburn, M., & Zhou, S. (2018). Technology-enhanced clinical simulations: Tools for practicing clinical skills in online social work programs. *Journal of Social Work Education, 54*(3), 554–560. http://dx.doi.org/10.1080/10437797.2017.1404519

Wittmann-Price, R., Godshall, M., & Wilson, L. (2017). *Certified Nurse Educator (CNE) review manual* (3rd ed.). Springer Publishing Company.

9

Competency-Based Education for Doctor of Nursing Practice (DNP) Curricula

Tracy P. George and Tiffany A. Phillips

"It is easier to do a job right than to explain why you didn't."

— Martin Van Buren

OBJECTIVES

- Define competency and competency-based education (CBE).
- Discuss how competencies have been integrated into graduate nursing curricula requirements.
- Describe the use of CBE in a Doctor of Nursing Practice (DNP) nursing curricula.

INTRODUCTION

Nurses enrolled in graduate programs must be prepared for their new roles when they complete their programs of study. Competency is what is needed to safely care for patients. "Although competency is defined in different ways, there is a common goal; to ensure nurses have the knowledge, skills, and abilities expected and required for their practice settings" (Anemia & McCoy, 2010, p. 6). In competency-based education (CBE), the nursing student must reach certain learning outcomes before advancing in their program (Gravina, 2017). CBE is aligned with the call for improved quality and safety in healthcare (Jamison & Lis, 2014).

In 2018, the National Organization of Nurse Practitioner Faculties (NONPF) called for the DNP degree to be the required entry-level degree for nurse practitioners (NP) by 2025, and many NP programs are moving toward the DNP as the entry-level degree. The purpose of the DNP is to equip nurses to "bridge the gap between the discovery of new knowledge and the scholarship of translation, application, and integration of this new knowledge in practice" (Waldrop et al., 2014, p. 300). NP students must attain competencies related to evidence-based practice to function in today's health system (Stiffler & Cullen, 2010).

NURSE PRACTITIONER CORE COMPETENCIES

BOX 9.1   EVIDENCE-BASED TEACHING PRACTICE

After validation by 31 participants, a competency-based formal transition into practice curriculum has been created for acute care NPs who are working in the intensive care unit (Kopf et al., 2018). This transition to practice competency-based curriculum incorporates the knowledge, skills, and attitudes for each competency topic (Kopf et al., 2018).

Competencies are important to NP education. The National Task Force on Quality Nurse Practitioner Education (NTF, 2016) developed the most recent version of the *Criteria for Evaluation of Nurse Practitioner Programs* in 2016. The NTF criteria, combined with accreditation standards, provide a foundation for evaluating all NP programs. According to Criterion VI.A.4 of the NTF, faculty are required to "evaluate students' attainment of competencies throughout the program," both in the didactic and clinical portions of content. For example, attainment of clinical competencies can be through clinical evaluations.

9.1 Example Vignette

The former clinical evaluation tool included ratings from the clinical preceptor at the end of the clinical experience. The areas of evaluation linked to the end-of-course student learning outcomes and did not always translate well to the clinical setting.

The tool was revised to allow for the evaluation of NONPF and NTF competencies specific to the clinical environment. The revision added midterm and final ratings by both the student and clinical preceptor, as well as midterm goals for the student for the remainder of the clinical experience. There are two versions of the clinical evaluation tool, one for BSN-DNP and BSN-MSN students and an abbreviated version for MSN-DNP students because they are already practicing as NPs.

Faculty need to ensure *Core Competencies for Nurse Practitioners* from NONPF are met (Levin & Suhayda, 2018). The NONPF competencies describe essential requirements for entry-level practice as an NP (LeCuyer et al., 2009). They are "guidelines not only for curriculum development but also for credentialing processes, clinical practice standards, and research" (LeCuyer et al., 2009, p. 186). The *Nurse Practitioner Core Competencies Content* was updated by NONPF in 2017 (NONPF, 2017b).

Faculty must incorporate the *Nurse Practitioner Core Competencies* into all NP and DNP courses, whether they are part of a BSN to MSN/FNP program, an MSN to DNP program, or a BSN to DNP program. The following includes each core competency with examples of specific assignments and/or curriculum content for each competency area.

NURSE PRACTITIONER CORE COMPETENCIES WITH EXAMPLES

Scientific Foundation

- Three P's: Advanced Pathophysiology, Advanced Pharmacology, Advanced Physical Assessment
- Development of PICOT (Population/Patient Problem, Intervention, Comparison, Outcome, Time) question to guide DNP Project
- Application of theoretical frameworks or quality improvement methods into the NP quality improvement projects and DNP projects

Leadership

- Leadership style analysis with discussion of strengths and weaknesses
- Discussion of change theories with application into mock quality improvement project early in curriculum
- Business plan development with inclusion of conflict and risk management strategies
- DNP manuscript preparation
- DNP poster development and presentation

Quality

- Outcomes of MSN and DNP projects evaluated
- Quality improvement methods discussed and incorporated into NP quality improvement and DNP projects
- Development of business plan with cost-benefit analysis

Practice Inquiry

- Use of PICOT model to guide literature search for best clinical evidence
- Use of library databases and clinical practice guidelines to guide decision-making in clinical, documentation, and case studies
- Reflective journals to identify gaps in patient care and treatment barriers
- Dissemination of work through DNP manuscript preparation and poster presentations
- Patient education articles submitted to local newspapers for publication
- Institutional and clinical site Institutional Review Board (IRB) approval required for DNP projects

Technology and Information Literacy

- Electronic databases available for use on smartphones or tablets in clinical
- Telehealth simulation incorporated into NP clinical course
- Patient portal discussion board incorporated into NP clinical course to simulate asynchronous telehealth
- Use of Centers for Disease Control and Prevention (CDC) datasets and County Health Rankings data to evaluate population health
- Objective Structured Clinical Examinations (OSCEs) in most NP clinical courses
- Use of health applications in clinical and OSCEs

Policy

- Barriers to NP practice discussion board
- Writing a letter to local legislators addressing current NP or health-related policy issue
- Attending state legislative day with faculty
- Global issues and social determinants of health incorporated into population health course through written assignments

Health Delivery System

- Evaluation of data to guide DNP project and improve practice
- Experience with e-prescribing during clinical
- Billing and coding principles discussed in clinical courses and evaluated in Typhon documentation
- Interprofessional topics including team building, collaboration, and conflict resolution incorporated through discussion boards

Ethics

- Institutional and Clinical site IRB approval required for DNP Project
- Advanced practice ethical issues with application of legal statutes and theories of ethical decision-making evaluated through written assignments

Independent Practice

- Clinical decision-making and the patient/provider partnership introduced through concepts of shared-decision aids and teach-back strategies
- Professional standards of practice evaluated through application of various scenarios in written assignments and OSCE and clinical evaluations
- Licensure, national certification, and scope of practice incorporated into discussion board assignments with comparisons of requirements of different states

- Credentialing and contract negotiation incorporated into on-site immersion experience
- Advanced health assessment course focused on varying assessment strategies for different populations
- Diagnostics incorporated into various clinical courses and OSCE and clinical evaluations
- Age- and gender-specific screening recommendations and health promotion strategies incorporated into all clinical courses and Typhon documentation
- Evidence-based pharmacologic recommendations incorporated into content of clinical courses, testing, OSCEs, and Typhon documentation
- Business plan development incorporated into risk management course

DOCTOR OF NURSING PRACTICE CORE COMPETENCIES

In 2017, NONPF released the *Common Advanced Practice Registered Nurse Doctoral-Level Competencies* (NONPF, 2017a), detailing eight observable and measurable domains. This document provides two progression times for evaluation during the program. Programs can use OSCEs with increasing complexity in most clinical courses, as well as midterm and final clinical self-assessments to evaluate many of the domains. Exhibit 9.1 includes each doctoral-level domain with examples of content for each domain.

Fast Facts

Interdisciplinary writing round tables are an excellent method to increase DNP students' writing competencies (Rohan & Fullerton, 2020).

Exhibit 9.1

Doctoral-Level Competencies with Examples

Domain	Examples of Curriculum Content
Patient Care: Designs, delivers, manages, and evaluates comprehensive patient care.	▪ Progression of OSCEs throughout the curriculum (see Example Vignette 9.1)
Knowledge of Practice: Synthesizes established and evolving scientific knowledge from diverse sources and contributes to the generation, translation, and dissemination of healthcare knowledge and practices.	▪ OSCE and Typhon evaluations demonstrate use of evidence to guide best practice on an individual level ▪ Literature synthesis, application of findings to clinical issue, and implementation and evaluation of DNP project reflect population focus
Practice-Based Learning & Improvement: Demonstrates the ability to investigate and evaluate one's care of patients, to appraise and assimilate emerging scientific evidence, and to continuously improve patient care based on constant self-evaluation and lifelong learning.	▪ Midterm and final self-evaluations as well as midterm clinical goals for the remainder of the clinical experience are required on the Clinical Evaluation Tool for all clinical courses ▪ Typhon documentation demonstrates use of current evidence-based practice by requiring a reference for each clinical encounter and an explanation for any portion of the treatment plan that does not follow current evidence-based practice recommendations ▪ DNP portfolio and curriculum vitae (CV) development emphasize involvement in lifelong learning ▪ Telehealth OSCE simulation focuses on emerging modalities to provide patient care

Interpersonal and Communication Skills: Demonstrates interpersonal and communication skills that result in the effective exchange of information and collaboration with patients, the public, and health professionals, and promote therapeutic relationships with patients across a broad range of cultural and socioeconomic backgrounds.

- OSCE scenarios include both straightforward sensitive issues with patients
- Telehealth OSCE and patient portal discussion board provide various ways in which technology can be used to provide patient care and exchange information

Professionalism: Demonstrates a commitment to carrying out professional responsibilities and an adherence to ethical principles.

- Various written assignments in courses taken during the first year of the curriculum focus on APRN scope of practice, philosophical frameworks, ethical principles, relevant laws and policies regulating the provision of care, health disparities, and health outcomes
- OSCE and clinical evaluations allow for direct evaluation of the delivery of compassionate, accountable care and application of ethical and moral principles
- Peer mentoring occurs during collaborative testing, group debriefing after the LGBTQ interviewing simulation in an advanced health assessment course, and the telehealth OSCE, which incorporates BSN students as the telehealth nurse
- DNP portfolio displays professional engagement of students
- DNP projects focus on improvement of healthcare outcomes

Systems-Based Practice: Demonstrates organizational and systems leadership to improve healthcare outcomes.

- Development of mock business plan early in curriculum explores cost-effectiveness and budgeting principles
- DNP project involves participation in quality improvement strategies
- Engagement with policymakers occurs through letter writing to legislators and participation in state-wide lobby day

(continued)

Exhibit 9.1

Doctoral-Level Competencies with Examples (*continued*)

Domain	Examples of Curriculum Content
Interprofessional Collaboration: Demonstrates the ability to engage in an interprofessional team in a manner that optimizes safe, effective patient- and population-centered care.	■ Evaluated in clinical courses through the clinical evaluation tool ■ DNP project requires leadership of an interprofessional team by the DNP student
Personal and Professional Development: Demonstrates the qualities required to sustain lifelong personal and professional growth.	■ The identification of their personal leadership style allows students to identify positives and negatives of their leadership style and consider strategies to address areas needing improvement

9.2 Example Vignette

OSCEs have been incorporated throughout the curriculum to allow faculty to observe and evaluate students' attainment of competencies. Early in the curriculum, OSCEs are straightforward and less complicated, focusing on episodic visits and common chronic disease management. OSCE content is varied with each clinical course to coincide with the course's populations and topics of focus. OSCEs have also allowed for the incorporation of telehealth simulation, sensitive topics, and prescription writing. The final OSCE evaluates the students' ability to evaluate, diagnose, and treat patients with multiple comorbidities.

SUMMARY

Assessment of competency ensures nursing graduates have the knowledge, skills, and abilities to practice in their specialty area. The National Task Force on Quality Nurse Practitioner Education (NTF, 2016) requires the evaluation of competencies throughout the curriculum of nurse practitioner programs. The National Organization of Nurse Practitioner Faculties (NONPF) has additionally identified competencies expected of the doctoral prepared advanced practice registered nurse. Since practice-based DNP programs are already required to meet core competencies for accreditation, it becomes a natural fit for these programs to employ competency-based education (CBE) in accomplishing this goal.

REFERENCES

Anemia, M., & McCoy, J. (2010). *Competency-based nursing education: Guide to achieving outstanding learner outcomes*. Springer Publishing Company.

Gravina, E. W. (2017). Competency-based education and its effect on nursing education: A literature review. *Teaching and Learning in Nursing, 12*(2), 117–121. http://dx.doi.org/10.1016/j.teln.2016.11.004

Jamison, T., & Lis, G. A. (2014). Engaging the learner by bridging the gap between theory and clinical competence. *Nursing Clinics of North America, 49*(1), 69–80. https://doi.org/10.4037/ajcc2018101

Kopf, R. S., Watts, P. I., Meyer, E. S., & Moss, J. A. (2018). A competency-based curriculum for critical care nurse practitioners' transition to practice. *American Journal of Critical Care, 27*(5), 398–406. https://doi.org/10.4037/ajcc2018101

LeCuyer, E., DeSocio, J., Brody, M., Schlick, R., & Menkens, R. (2009). From objectives to competencies: Operationalizing the NONPF PMHNP competencies for use in a graduate curriculum. *Archives of Psychiatric Nursing, 23*(3), 185–199. http://dx.doi.org/10.1016/j.apnu.2008.06.004

Levin, P. F., & Suhayda, R. (2018). Transitioning to the DNP: Ensuring integrity of the curriculum through curriculum mapping. *Nurse Educator, 43*(3), 112–114. http://dx.doi.org/10.1097/NNE.0000000000000431

National Organization of Nurse Practitioner Faculties. (2017a). *Common advanced practice registered nurse doctoral-level competencies.* https://cdn.ymaws.com/www.nonpf.org/resource/resmgr/competencies/common-aprn-sdoctoral-compete.pdf

National Organization of Nurse Practitioner Faculties. (2017b). *Nurse practitioner core competencies content.* https://cdn.ymaws.com/www.nonpf.org/resource/resmgr/competencies/2017_NPCoreCosmps_with_Curric.pdf

National Organization of Nurse Practitioner Faculties. (2018). *The doctor of nursing practice degree: Entry to nurse practitioner practice by 2025.* https://cdn.ymaws.com/www.nonpf.org/resource/resmgr/dnp/v3_05.2018_NONPF_DNPStateme.pdf

National Task Force on Quality Nurse Practitioner Education. (2016). *Criteria for evaluation of nurse practitioner programs* (5th ed.). https://cdn.ymaws.com/www.nonpf.org/resource/resmgr/Docs/EvalCriteria2016Final.pdf

Rohan, A., & Fullerton, J. (2020). Interdisciplinary peer mentorship: An innovative strategy to enhance writing competency. *Journal of Nursing Education, 59*(3), 173–175. https://doi.org/10.3928/01484834-20200220-11

Stiffler, D., & Cullen, D. (2010). Evidence-based practice for nurse practitioner students: A competency-based teaching framework. *Journal of Professional Nursing, 26*(5), 272–277. http://dx.doi .org/10.1016/j.profnurs.2010.02.004

Waldrop, J., Caruso, D., Fuchs, M. A., & Hypes, K. (2014). EC as pie: Five criteria for executing a successful DNP final. *Journal of Professional Nursing, 30*(4), 300–306. http://dx.doi.org/10.1016/ j.profnurs.2014.01.003

Index

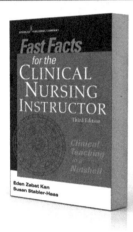
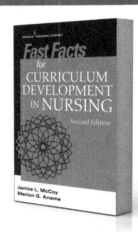
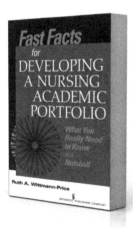
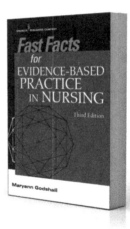

Printed in the United States
by Baker & Taylor Publisher Services